Neuro-Ophthalmology:
A Problem-Oriented Approach

Neuro-Ophthalmology:
A Problem-Oriented Approach

Roy W. Beck, M.D.

ASSOCIATE PROFESSOR OF OPHTHALMOLOGY, NEUROLOGY, AND NEUROSURGERY
AND DIRECTOR, NEURO-OPHTHALMOLOGY SERVICE,
UNIVERSITY OF SOUTH FLORIDA COLLEGE OF MEDICINE,
TAMPA, FLORIDA

Craig H. Smith, M.D.

CLINICAL ASSOCIATE PROFESSOR OF MEDICINE (NEUROLOGY) AND OPHTHALMOLOGY,
UNIVERSITY OF WASHINGTON SCHOOL OF MEDICINE;
DIRECTOR, EYE INSTITUTE OF SWEDISH HOSPITAL MEDICAL CENTER,
SEATTLE, WASHINGTON

Little, Brown and Company
Boston Toronto

To our wives,
Ruth and Sharon,
and our children,
Jody, Andy, Eric, and Galen

Contents

Preface

1. *The Neuro-Ophthalmic Examination 1*
2. *Optic Neuritis 34*
3. *Optic Neuritis in a Child 42*
4. *Anterior Ischemic Optic Neuropathy 46*
5. *Giant Cell Arteritis 53*
6. *Pseudotumor Cerebri 58*
7. *Pseudopapilledema 66*
8. *Compressive Optic Neuropathy 73*
9. *Optic Glioma 80*
10. *Hereditary Optic Atrophy 84*
11. *Leber's Optic Neuropathy 88*
12. *Nutritional Optic Neuropathy 92*
13. *Traumatic Optic Neuropathy 98*
14. *Optic Nerve Hypoplasia 102*
15. *Amaurosis Fugax 106*
16. *Uncommon Optic Neuropathies 111*
17. *Chiasmal Syndrome—Pituitary Tumor 122*
18. *Optic Tract Syndrome 132*
19. *Homonymous Hemianopia 136*
20. *Migraine 144*
21. *Functional Visual Loss 148*
22. *Limited Upgaze—Graves' Ophthalmopathy 153*
23. *Fourth Nerve Palsy 163*
24. *Third Nerve Palsy 168*
25. *Dorsal Midbrain Syndrome 179*
26. *Skew Deviation 184*
27. *Sixth Nerve Palsy 188*
28. *Internuclear Ophthalmoplegia 197*
29. *Fisher's Syndrome 205*
30. *Orbital Apex Syndrome 216*
31. *Myasthenia Gravis 221*
32. *Lid Retraction 232*
33. *Horner's Syndrome 234*
34. *Dilated Pupil—Adie's Syndrome 239*
35. *Cavernous Sinus Fistula 245*
36. *Essential Blepharospasm 253*

Index 261

Preface

Neuro-ophthalmology is a discipline comprising a multitude of disorders that overlap the fields of ophthalmology, neurology, and general medicine. Diagnosis in this field is frequently a challenge even for the neuro-ophthalmologist. Proper management rests in the ability to formulate a differential diagnosis from the patient's history and examination findings. Far too often clinicians substitute x-rays and other ancillary tests for a proper neuro-ophthalmic examination in an attempt to reach a diagnosis.

This book provides a broad overview of neuro-ophthalmology. It uses case studies, stressing the fundamentals of the neuro-ophthalmic examination, to develop a foundation of neuro-ophthalmic principles. We hope that it will provide a set of ground rules that will facilitate diagnosis and improve patient care.

The major thrust of the book is clinical neuro-ophthalmology. We have chosen topics that we feel represent the entities most commonly encountered by the clinician and have presented each in the form of a case history with a subsequent discussion. Each case consists of the patient's history and pertinent physical findings including visual fields and photographs of the fundus or eye movements when appropriate.* The material following presents a differential diagnosis and a practical clinical discussion of the topic including the proper management and the prognosis.

Neuro-ophthalmology is a complicated subject that can be difficult to grasp. We think that the presentation of material in the form of cases is an excellent method by which to master this field. This book should be of interest to ophthalmologists, neurologists, and neurosurgeons, as well as to residents in these fields.

R. W. B.
C. H. S.

*Slides of the cases presented in this book may be purchased by contacting Craig H. Smith, M.D., Nordstrom Medical Tower, 1229 Madison, Suite 1490, Seattle, WA 98104.

Neuro-Ophthalmology:
A Problem-Oriented Approach

1

The Neuro-Ophthalmic Examination

A properly performed history and examination are essential to diagnosing neuro-ophthalmic disorders correctly. Too often a laboratory or neuroradiologic investigation is undertaken before a sufficient examination, and only after the results are unenlightening is a proper neuro-ophthalmic evaluation performed.

In this chapter we review certain aspects of the neuro-ophthalmic examination as well as the clinical approach to diagnosing common neuro-ophthalmic disorders.

Evaluation of Visual Function

VISUAL ACUITY

Visual acuity may be reduced with optic nerve, chiasmal, or optic tract lesions, but it is never affected by unilateral retrogeniculate lesions.

In assessing visual function, one is interested in the patient's vision with the best possible refractive correction (called *best corrected vision*). Thus, a patient should wear his or her glasses for the test. Ideally a refraction should be performed to determine the best corrected acuity, but for the neurologist, this is not possible. Whenever visual acuity is reduced, a pinhole should be tried. This device, by reducing the size of the blur circle on the retina, will improve visual acuity in an eye with an uncorrected refractive error, but because of the diffraction it produces, 20/25 is frequently the best acuity that can be obtained. With proper refraction, visual acuity usually is equal at distance and near; a discrepancy between the two measurements suggests that an uncorrected refractive error is present.

The standard of vision testing is the Snellen eye chart. Visual acuity is recorded as a fraction, with the numerator being the testing distance and the denominator being the distance at which the letter subtends an angle of 1 minute of arc. Thus, 20/20 acuity means that at 20 ft, a letter subtending an angle of 1 minute of arc can be identified. A 20/40 letter on the chart is twice the size of a 20/20 letter; a 20/200 letter is 10 times the size. If the patient cannot identify the 20/400 letter, he or she is moved closer to the chart and the visual acuity is recorded accordingly. If the patient can identify the letter at 5 ft, for instance, the acuity is 5/400. When no letters on the chart can be identified, the ability to count fingers, see a hand moving, or appreciate a light shined on the eye is determined. Finger counting at 10 ft approximates 20/200 vision.

In infants, vision is assessed by judging how well the baby fixates on and follows an object. In young infants, the human face is a good visual stimulus to employ. As a child gets older, he or she can be asked to identify pictures, or the illiterate E chart may be used.

COLOR VISION

Although dyschromatopsia may occur with a lesion in most portions of the visual system, testing of color vision is most useful in assessing optic nerve function. Perception of color tends to be impaired earlier with an optic neuropathy than with a maculopathy. Severe monocular dyschromatopsia with only minimal reduction in visual acuity supports an optic nerve cause of visual loss. Normal color vision with acuity reduced to 20/100 or less suggests that visual loss is not neurogenic.

Color plates (such as Ishihara or Hardy-Rand-Rittler tests) provide a simple, fast method of assessing color vision. In interpreting the results it must be remembered that approximately 8 percent of males and 0.5 percent of females have an inherited X-linked recessive congenital color deficiency. Each eye must be tested separately. A score can be assigned to each eye based on the number of plates correctly identified. Any differences between the two eyes either in the number of plates correctly identified or the speed in responding should be considered abnormal.

Since most acquired optic neuropathies do not produce a specific axis of color deficit, more sophisticated testing of color vision is usually not necessary. In suspected cases of hereditary optic atrophy, however, identification of a yellow-blue deficiency will assist in diagnosis (see Chapter 10). The Farnsworth-Munsell 15-hue or 100-hue test is the most available test of this type.

A subjective assessment of color perception can be obtained by having the patient compare the brightness of a colored object viewed alternately with each eye. A desaturated appearance of the color in one eye compared to the other suggests an optic nerve cause of visual loss.

AFFERENT PUPILLARY REACTION

The assessment of the pupillary reaction is the only completely objective test of visual function. When performed properly, it provides an indication of the integrity of the visual system from the retina through the optic tract. Before the reactivity to light is assessed, pupillary size should be recorded under both bright and dim illuminations. The evaluation of anisocoria is described later in this chapter.

Certain points about the technique of testing the pupillary light reflex deserve emphasis. First, room illumination must be low. The darker the examination room, the larger the pupils will be and the more easily a subtle difference in reaction between the pupils will be detected. Second, the patient must be instructed to fixate in the distance. If distance fixation is not maintained, particularly if the patient looks at the light directed at the eye, the pupils will constrict as part of the near response, and the light reflex cannot be assessed. In infants and children, it is often difficult to eliminate this response completely, and thus subtle differ-

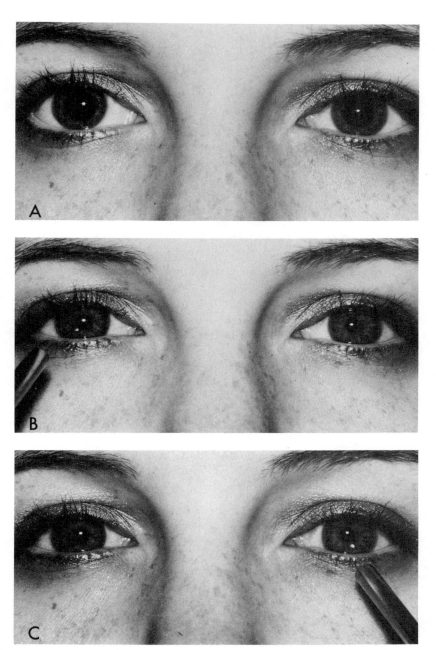

Fig. 1-1.
Testing for a relative afferent pupillary defect (normal subject). A. With diffuse illumination pupils are of equal size. B. With light on right eye, both pupils constrict. C. They remain constricted when light is swung to left eye. (From C. H. Smith and R. W. Beck. The neuro-ophthalmic examination. Neurol. Clin. 1:807, 1983. Reprinted with permission from W. B. Saunders Co.)

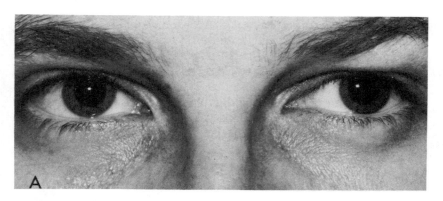

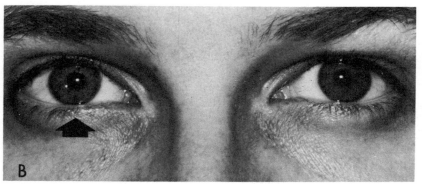

ences between the pupillary reaction in each eye may be missed. Third, a bright flashlight should be used. The brighter the light, the more a relative difference in the transmission of light through the afferent pathway of the two eyes will be apparent.

Alternating Light Test. The alternating light (Marcus-Gunn) test assesses the afferent arc of the pupillary light reflex pathway [2]. In simple terms, the test is a comparison of the direct and consensual response to light in each eye. Since the two responses are normally essentially equal, any difference between them (assuming an intact efferent arc) is indicative of a relative afferent pupillary defect. A relative afferent pupillary defect may be detectable with a lesion in the retina, optic nerve, optic chiasm, or optic tract but not one further posterior in the visual system.

The technique for the alternating light test is described in Figs. 1-1 and 1-2. With a large defect in the afferent arc, a relative afferent pupillary defect will be obvious. With a slight impairment, it may be very subtle, and the first movement of the pupil may still be one of constriction. This is because of the enhanced retinal sensitivity in the eye in relative darkness compared to the eye on which the light is shined. However, if the pupil is observed for 1 to 2 seconds, it will be seen to dilate after the initial constriction, whereas when the light is swung to the pupil of the normal eye, it constricts and remains so.

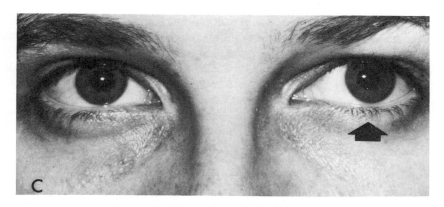

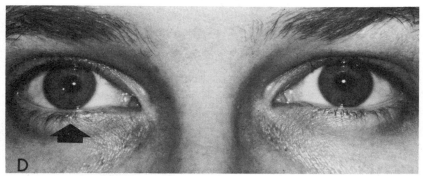

Fig. 1-2.
Testing for a relative afferent pupillary defect in a patient with a left optic neuropathy. (Arrows indicate eye on which bright light is directed.) A. With diffuse illumination, pupils are of equal size. B. With light on right eye, pupils constrict briskly. C. Pupils dilate slightly when light is swung to left eye. D. When light is swung back to right eye, both pupils constrict to the size they were in B. (From C. H. Smith and R. W. Beck. The neuro-ophthalmic examination. Neurol. Clin. 1:807, 1983. Reprinted with permission from W. B. Saunders Co.)

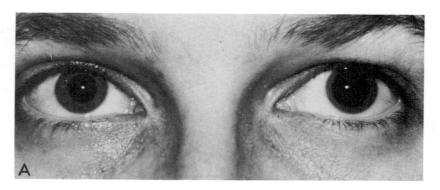

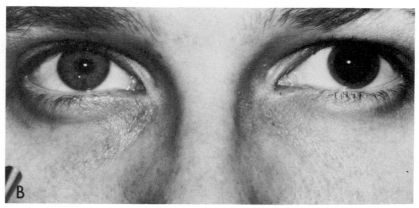

When the pupil of one eye is unreactive because of an efferent problem (e.g., third nerve palsy, traumatic iridoplegia, or pharmacologic iridoplegia), the alternating light test can still be performed with all observations being made on the reactive pupil (Fig. 1-3).

Remember that the alternating light test detects only a relative difference between the afferent pupillary reaction in the two eyes. Thus, with equal loss of visual field in both eyes, as with many bilateral optic neuropathies or chiasmal lesions, a relative afferent pupillary defect will not be apparent.

A relative afferent pupillary defect can be quantitated by using neutral density filters [3]. Filters of increasing density are placed before the "normal" eye until the pupillary responses appear equal in the alternating light test (Fig. 1-4). The filter is also of benefit in cases in which a relative afferent pupillary defect is equivocal. A neutral density filter placed first in front of one eye and then the other during the alternating light test should produce a symmetric response. If not, a slight difference in pupillary response between the two eyes can be inferred.

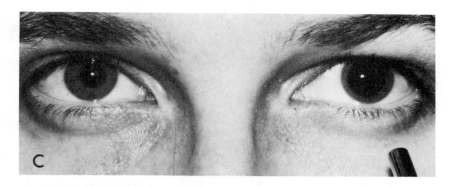

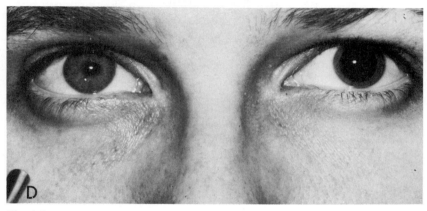

Fig. 1-3.
Testing for a relative afferent pupillary defect when one pupil is dilated. A left optic neuropathy is present. A. With diffuse illumination left pupil is larger than right. B. With light on right eye, right pupil constricts but left does not. C. When light is swung to left eye, right pupil dilates slightly. D. Pupil again constricts when light is swung back to right eye. (From C. H. Smith and R. W. Beck. The neuro-ophthalmic examination. Neurol. Clin. 1:807, 1983. Reprinted with permission from W. B. Saunders Co.)

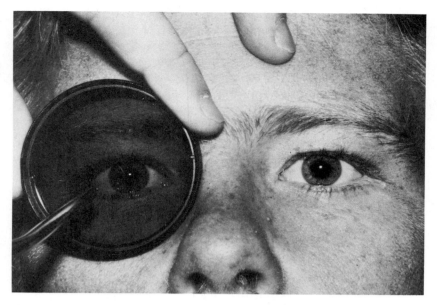

Fig. 1-4.
A neutral density filter held in front of the right eye during the alternating light test to neutralize a relative afferent pupillary defect present in left eye. (From C. H. Smith and R. W. Beck. The neuro-ophthalmic examination. Neurol. Clin. *1:807, 1983. Reprinted with permission from W. B. Saunders Co.)*

VISUAL FIELD

Assessing the visual field is an essential part of the examination of the afferent visual system. The pattern of visual field loss will indicate not only which portion of the visual system is most likely to be involved but also the most likely causes. Terms commonly used to describe visual field defects are defined in the following list:

Isopter   the extent of the visual field that is plotted with a given stimulus.
Homonymous   affecting the same side of the visual field in each eye.
Heteronymous   affecting the opposite side of the visual field in each eye.
Congruity   the degree of correspondence of the visual field loss in each eye with a homonymous defect.
Depression   a relative loss of visual field, that is, some stimuli are seen while others are not.
Contraction   absolute loss of visual field, usually peripheral, such that no stimuli are seen in the affected area.
Scotoma   an abnormal area of visual field surrounded by normal visual field. A scotoma is called *absolute* when no stimuli are perceived in the area and *relative* when some stimuli are appreciated while others are not.
Macular sparing   homonymous visual field defects in which the macular representation on the involved side is wholly or in part unaffected.

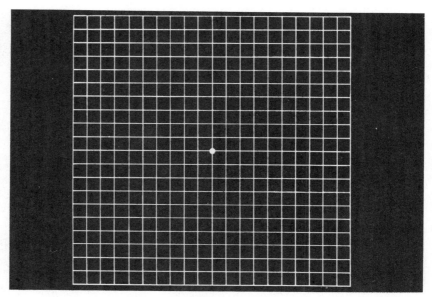

Fig. 1-5.
Amsler grid. The patient views the grid monocularly. Any distorted, blurred, or missing areas in the grid are marked. (From C. H. Smith and R. W. Beck. The neuro-ophthalmic examination. Neurol. Clin. 1:807, 1983. Reprinted with permission from W. B. Saunders Co.)

Temporal crescent   the peripheral portion of the temporal visual field that has only monocular representation in the occipital lobe.

Nerve fiber bundle defect   a visual field defect, occurring with either a retinal or optic nerve lesion, that follows a pattern of loss of nerve fibers. Examples include nasal arcuate scotomas, steps and altitudinal defects, and temporal sector defects.

Visual field testing can be performed by several methods: Amsler grid, confrontation techniques, perimetry, and tangent screen.

Amsler Grid. The central 10 degrees of the field (10 degrees in all directions from fixation) can be assessed subjectively with an Amsler grid (Fig. 1-5). The test is particularly useful when the patient complains of metamorphopsia and reports a distorted area of central visual field but is also useful in detecting central and paracentral scotomas.

Confrontation Techniques. Confrontation visual field testing yields an enormous amount of information and when performed properly on a cooperative patient will detect most visual field defects. There are numerous methods that may be used, but we describe in Fig. 1-6 steps we have found useful.

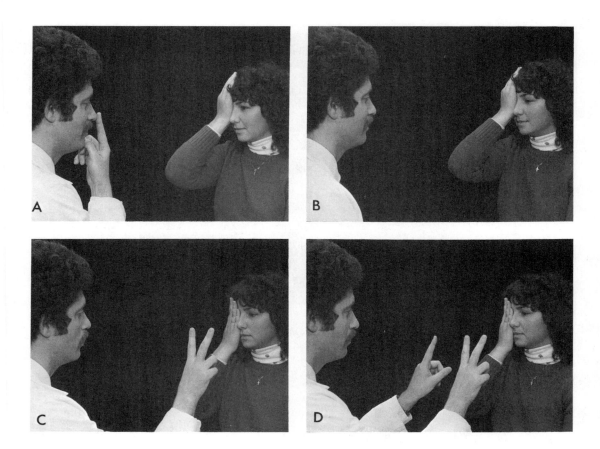

Note that unless we suspect a severe generalized constriction of the visual field, we do not routinely bring a moving target, such as our hands, in from the side to assess the absolute extent of the field. This technique will not detect a relative field defect and only rarely will provide information not obtained with the technique that is illustrated.

When the visual field is constricted and malingering or hysteria is suspected, it is useful to perform confrontation testing at various distances to see if the visual field appropriately expands and contracts.

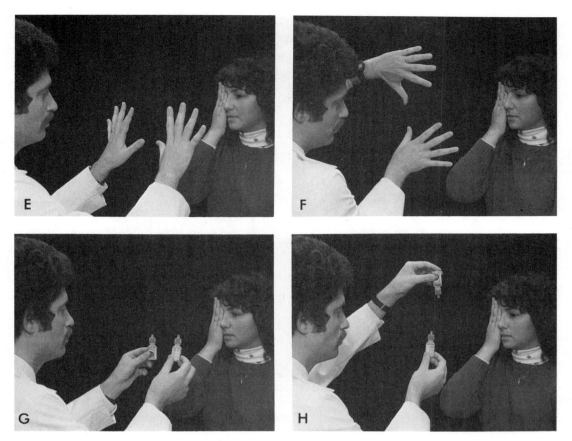

Fig. 1-6.
Confrontation visual field technique. Each eye is tested separately. A. The patient is instructed to maintain fixation on the examiner's nose throughout the test. The patient is asked the questions in B through H. B. Does the examiner's face appear clear, or are there gaps or blurred areas? This tests the central few degrees of the field. C, D. Count fingers in each quadrant separately (C) and then simultaneously (D) on each side of the vertical meridian. If the fingers in a given area cannot be identified the patient is asked whether hand movement can be, and the abnormal area is mapped out by moving the hand until a normal area is reached. E, F. Compare the clarity of the examiner's hands, which are placed on each side of the vertical meridian in first the upper and then the lower quadrants (E) and then above and below the horizontal meridian on each side (F). If an abnormal area is detected, the hand is moved until it appears clear. G, H. Compare the color of two red targets (such as the tops of mydriatic drop bottles) placed simultaneously on each side of the vertical meridian in first the upper and then the lower quadrants (G) and then above and below the horizontal meridian on each side (H). If one appears desaturated compared with the other, it is moved to map out the abnormal area. Occasionally the patient may consider the red target in a defective area to be the better color since a deeper red may be interpreted as being better than a more orange red. (From C. H. Smith and R. W. Beck. The neuro-ophthalmic examination. Neurol. Clin. 1:807, 1983. Reprinted with permission from W. B. Saunders Co.)

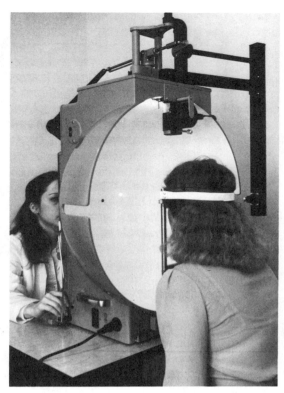

Fig. 1-7.
Goldmann perimeter. The patient is on the right; the perimetrist, on the left. (From C. H. Smith and R. W. Beck. The neuro-ophthalmic examination. Neurol. Clin. *1:807, 1983. Reprinted with permission from W. B. Saunders Co.)*

Perimetry. Spherical projection perimetry (Goldmann equivalent) has become the standard of visual field testing (Fig. 1-7). Although great strides have been made in the development of automated perimetry, the Goldmann perimeter has not yet been supplanted and may never be. With this instrument the visual field can be plotted accurately either kinetically or statically with a high degree of reproducibility. Having an expensive, well-calibrated instrument, however, without a well-trained perimetrist is nonproductive and will result in inadequate visual field assessment. Trobe and associates found that community-based perimetrists had little understanding of the basic principles of perimetry and that their visual field plottings were generally unreliable [4]. Thus a visual field is only as good as the perimetrist who plots it.

Automated perimetry is playing an ever-increasing role in the evaluation of visual field defects. Although many instruments are now available, perimeters that measure the light threshold at various points in the visual field hold the greatest promise. With an instrument that performs static perimetry, visual field defects not disclosed with standard testing

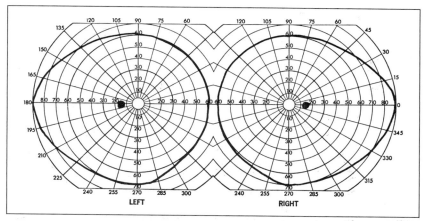

Fig. 1-8.
The extent of the normal visual field. (From C. H. Smith and R. W. Beck. The neuro-ophthalmic examination. Neurol. Clin. 1:807, 1983. Reprinted with permission from W. B. Saunders Co.)

on the Goldmann perimeter may be detectable. This is particularly true in cases of glaucoma, but in most neuro-ophthalmic disorders manual kinetic testing is generally of comparable sensitivity.

Tangent Screen. When a perimeter is unavailable, a tangent screen may be used to plot the visual field. Although only the central 25 degrees of the visual field can be tested, most lesions, whether in the optic nerve, chiasm, or retrochiasmal visual system, produce some degree of depression of the central field. Thus, although an absolute peripheral defect may be missed, a central depression will be plotted.

The tangent screen plays a major role in the analysis of the functional visual field, since the distance from the patient to the screen can be varied.

Principals of Visual Field Interpretation. The normal visual field extends approximately 100 degrees temporally, 60 degrees nasally, 60 degrees superiorly, and 70 degrees inferiorly (Fig. 1-8). The physiologic blind spot can be plotted approximately 15 degrees temporal to fixation and generally extends slightly further inferiorly than superiorly. The central visual field consists of the area within 30 degrees of fixation; the area outside this is called the peripheral visual field.

In anatomic localization of visual field defects, we have found several steps useful. To start, we determine whether the defects are in one or both eyes. Visual field defects affecting only one eye indicate retinal or optic nerve pathology. These defects may obey the horizontal meridian but almost never respect the vertical. If the defects are in both eyes, we determine whether they are homonymous or heteronymous and whether they respect the vertical meridian. Binasal visual field defects

Table 1-1. Localization of lesions in the visual system

Parameter	Optic nerve	Optic chiasm	Optic tract	Temporal lobe	Parietal lobe	Occipital lobe
Visual acuity	Normal or reduced	Normal or reduced	Normal or reduced	Normal	Normal	Normal
Color vision	Normal or reduced	Normal or reduced	Normal or reduced	Normal	Normal	Normal
Visual field	Central scotoma Nerve fiber bundle defect	Bitemporal	Homonymous, incongruous	Homonymous, superior	Homonymous, inferior or complete	Homonymous, exquisitely congruous
RAPD	+	±	±	−	−	−
Disk pallor	±	±	±	−	−	−

Key: RAPD = relative afferent pupillary defect; + = present; − = absent.

indicate bilateral optic nerve disease (see differential diagnosis of nerve fiber bundle defects on page 16) whereas bitemporal defects that extend to, but not beyond, the vertical meridian implicate the optic chiasm as the site of pathology. A homonymous hemianopia may occur with a lesion in the optic tract, lateral geniculate body, optic radiations, or occipital lobe. Assessment of visual acuity, pupillary reaction, congruity, and the optokinetic response may be helpful in localization. Table 1-1 summarizes the approach to localization of a deficit within the visual system.

Common Disorders of the Afferent Visual System
OPTIC NERVE DISORDERS
Localization of a visual disturbance to the optic nerve can almost always be made on examination based on visual acuity, color vision, pupillary reactions, and the visual field. A differential diagnosis for the cause of the optic neuropathy in a given patient can be established by categorizing the patient on the basis of the pattern of visual field loss, the optic disk appearance, and whether one or both eyes are involved.

Visual Field Defects. Visual field defects from optic neuropathies follow several patterns. It is useful to classify the disorders into those that tend to produce central or cecocentral scotomas and those that produce nerve fiber bundle field defects.

A central scotoma occurs when a lesion involves the papillomacular bundle (Fig. 1-9). The cause of a unilateral central scotoma is generally different from that of bilateral central scotomas. A unilateral central scotoma is most commonly due to optic neuritis or a compressive lesion. A history of sudden visual loss suggests the former; a history of slowly progressive visual loss suggests the latter. With a unilateral central scotoma, it is extremely important to assess the visual field in the fellow eye

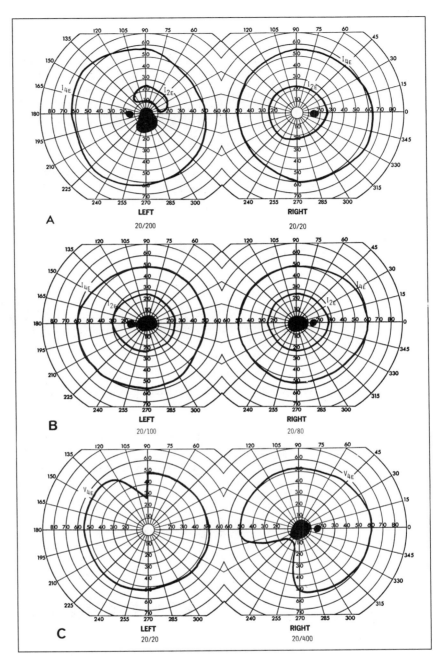

Fig. 1-9.
A. Unilateral central scotoma in a patient with optic neuritis. B. Bilateral central scotoma in a patient with nutritional optic neuropathy. C. Anterior junctional syndrome from compression of the right optic nerve anterior to the optic chiasm by a meningioma. Note superior temporal defect in left eye, which localizes the disease to the posterior optic nerve. (From C. H. Smith and R. W. Beck. The neuro-ophthalmic examination. Neurol. Clin. 1:807, 1983. Reprinted with permission from W. B. Saunders Co.)

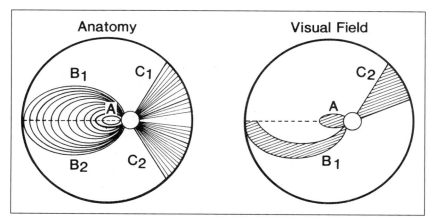

Fig. 1-10.
Distribution of retinal nerve fibers as they enter the optic nerve.

for the presence of a temporal defect, which would indicate involvement of the posterior optic nerve and chiasm and make a compressive lesion likely (see Chapters 2 and 8). Bilateral central scotomas are generally the result of poor nutrition (tobacco-alcohol amblyopia), drugs, toxins, hereditary optic atrophy, or, less commonly, infiltration of the optic nerves, bilateral compressive lesions, or optic neuritis.

Several disorders that affect the optic nerve at the level of the optic disk spare the papillomacular bundle and produce what are called *nerve fiber bundle defects* (Figs. 1-10, 1-11). These defects may take several forms, but they all have a pattern mimicking the distribution of the nerve fibers in the retina, with respect to the horizontal but not the vertical meridian. The fibers from the temporal retina are affected much more commonly than the fibers from the nasal retina, presumably because of their anatomic distribution within the optic nerve. Since the papillomacular bundle occupies much of the temporal portion of the optic disk, the fibers from the temporal retina are "squeezed" into the superior and inferior poles. Nerve fiber bundle defects occur with glaucoma, optic nerve drusen, chronic papilledema, ischemic optic neuropathy, and branch retinal artery occlusion. Visual acuity is often normal in all of these entities.

Optic Disk Appearance. With an optic neuropathy the optic disk may appear normal, swollen, or pale. Table 1-2 provides a differential diagnosis based on the appearance of the disk.

Swollen Optic Disk. In assessing a swollen optic disk, a determination should first be made as to whether there is acquired disk edema or whether the disk appearance is that of pseudopapilledema. This distinction can almost always be made on the basis of the ophthalmoscopic findings (see Chapter 7).

If it is determined that true disk edema is present, it is useful to sepa-

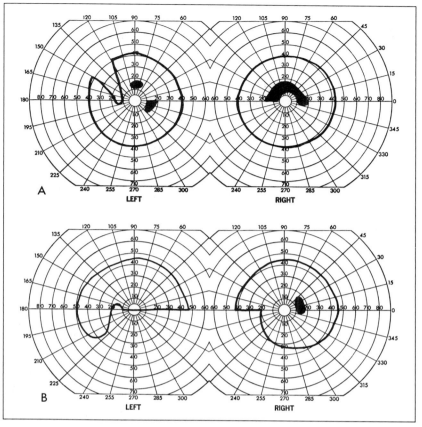

Fig. 1-11.
Nerve fiber bundle defects. A. In the right eye an arcuate scotoma is present. In the left there is a scotoma in the Bjerrum area and a temporal sector defect. Note how the inferior scotoma obeys the horizontal meridian. B. A nasal step is present in the right eye, an inferior altitudinal defect in the left eye. (From C. H. Smith and R. W. Beck. The neuro-ophthalmic examination. Neurol. Clin. 1:807, 1983. Reprinted with permission from W. B. Saunders Co.)

rate cases into unilateral and bilateral categories and further subdivide them as to whether optic nerve function is normal or impaired.

The most common causes of unilateral optic disk edema are optic neuritis, anterior ischemic optic neuropathy, and orbital tumors. Optic nerve function will as a rule be abnormal in each. Although it may be impossible to distinguish these entities by the optic disk appearance, diagnosis can usually be established based on the history of visual loss and the pattern of visual field deficit. As is demonstrated in Fig. 1-12, visual loss is generally slowly progressive with compressive lesions, sudden with subsequent improvement in optic neuritis, and sudden without improvement in ischemic optic neuropathy.

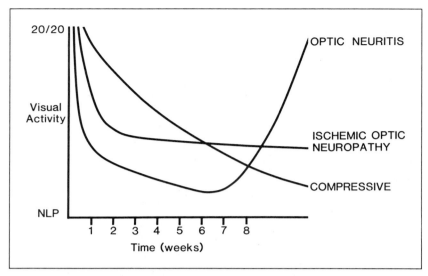

Fig. 1-12.
Time course of visual loss in optic neuritis, anterior ischemic optic neuropathy, and compressive optic neuropathy. Key: NLP = no light perception.

Less common causes of unilateral disk edema include obstruction of the central retinal vein and infiltrative disorders. Optic nerve function is generally normal in the former and impaired in the latter. In extremely rare circumstances, papilledema (from increased intracranial pressure) occurs unilaterally.

Bilateral optic disk edema is usually due to increased intracranial pressure and in this setting is called *papilledema*. Optic nerve function is typically normal in papilledema. Malignant hypertension could produce a similar picture. Any of the entities producing unilateral disk edema can occasionally occur in a bilateral form.

Table 1-2. *Causes of optic neuropathy categorized by optic disk appearance*

Edema		Normal		Atrophy	
Unilateral	Bilateral	Unilateral	Bilateral	Cupped	Not cupped
Optic neuritis	Papilledema	Retrobulbar	Tobacco-alcohol	Glaucoma	Any optic
Ischemic optic	(increased	neuritis	amblyopia	Giant cell	neuropathy
neuropathy	intracranial	Compressive	Nutritional	arteritis	
Orbital tumor	pressure)	lesion	Drugs		
Other: papillo-	Malignant	Infiltration:	Toxins		
phlebitis,	hypertension	granulomatous,	Hereditary*		
central retinal	Diabetic	carcinomatous,	Any of the		
vein occlusion,	papillopathy	lymphomatous	unilateral		
infiltrative	Any of the		causes		
disorders	unilateral				
	causes				

*Optic disk may appear swollen acutely in Leber's optic neuropathy.

Table 1-3. *Differentiation of optic nerve and macular disease*

Parameter	Optic nerve	Macula
Visual acuity	Reduced	Reduced
Color vision	Impaired	Preserved
Visual field	Central scotoma	Normal or small central scotoma
Pupils	RAPD	Normal
Photostress test	Normal	Abnormal
Light brightness sense	Reduced	Normal

Key: RAPD = relative afferent pupillary defect.

Optic Neuropathies with a Normal Optic Disk. In many types of optic neuropathy, the optic disk may appear completely normal. In these cases, misdiagnosis or delay in diagnosis is all too common. Differentiation of optic nerve and macular disease is summarized in Table 1-3. This table is meant to provide guidelines and not absolute conditions.

Two of the tests cited in the table deserve further mention. The photostress test described by Glaser and associates consists of shining a bright light into first one and then the other eye and recording the amount of time that elapses before visual acuity in each eye recovers to its level before the test [1]. In the presence of macular disease, recovery of vision after light stimulation may be prolonged because of the delay in the photochemical processes that occur after the retina is bleached with light. With optic nerve disease, the recovery time should be normal.

A comparison of light brightness sense between the two eyes may also help differentiate visual loss owing to an optic nerve disorder from visual loss of macular origin. A bright light is shone first in one eye and then the other, and the patient is asked whether one appears brighter than the other. With an optic neuropathy, light sensitivity tends to be reduced, whereas with macular lesions it does not.

Most retrobulbar optic neuropathies produce a central scotoma in the visual field. The differential diagnosis is different for unilateral and bilateral cases. In unilateral cases, a compressive lesion or retrobulbar neuritis is the most likely cause. As discussed previously, the history of visual loss is usually helpful in distinguishing the two. There is no definite way to distinguish them on examination, but detection of a superotemporal visual field defect in the fellow eye would be highly suggestive of a compressive lesion. The most common masses affecting the optic nerve are meningioma, pituitary tumor, craniopharyngioma, aneurysm, and mucocele. Gliomas are common in children but rare in adults.

Bilateral optic neuropathies in which the optic disk appears normal include nutritional optic neuropathy (tobacco-alcohol amblyopia), vitamin B_{12} or folate deficiencies, toxic neuropathy (in particular, from heavy metals), and drug-related neuropathy (from chloramphenicol, isoniazid, ethambutol, ethchlorvynol [Placidyl], chlorpropamide, and others). When these conditions are chronic, optic atrophy may ensue.

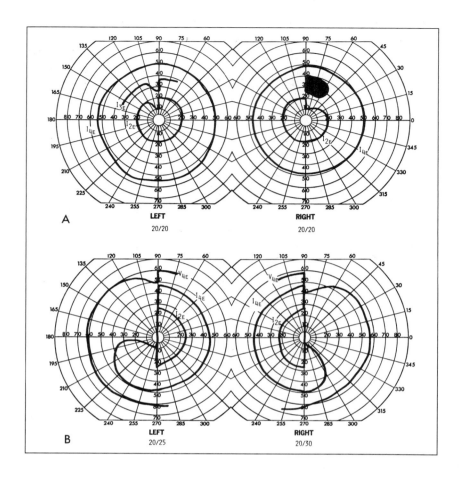

Other diagnostic considerations in this category include an inherited optic atrophy, bilateral compressive lesions, and bilateral optic neuritis.

Optic Atrophy. Any optic neuropathy may result in optic atrophy. At this stage the optic disk appearance is frequently not helpful in determining the underlying cause, although the presence of gliosis suggests that the disk was previously swollen, and acquired cupping is most typical of either glaucoma or temporal arteritis. Optic atrophy is also a possible consequence of lesions in the retina, optic chiasm, and optic tract.

Optic Chiasm

The fibers from the nasal retina cross in the optic chiasm, with the fibers from the inferior nasal retina crossing first and passing slightly forward in the contralateral optic nerve (Wilbrandt's knee) before proceeding posteriorly. Thus a lesion of the posterior optic nerve produces a central scotoma in the homolateral eye and a superior temporal field defect in the contralateral eye. As was previously mentioned, a compressive lesion is the usual cause. Lesions of the chiasm itself produce temporal visual

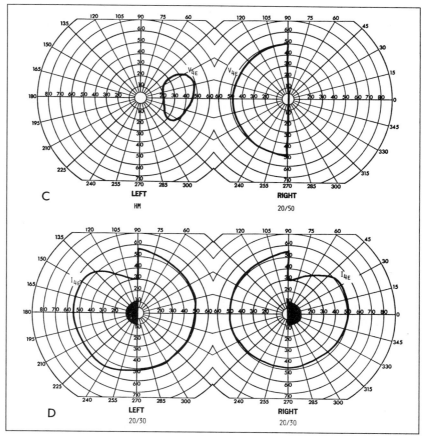

Fig. 1-13.

Examples of visual field loss with chiasmal lesion. A, B. Note that the defects are relative. C. The defects are absolute. D. Note the bitemporal defect involving both the macular and peripheral fibers. (From C. H. Smith and R. W. Beck. The neuro-ophthalmic examination. Neurol. Clin. 1:807, 1983. Reprinted with permission from W. B. Saunders Co.)

field loss in both eyes that typically obeys the vertical meridian in at least one eye. The field loss may take many forms, with central or peripheral involvement predominating (Fig. 1-13). If the fibers subserving macular vision are involved, reduced visual acuity, dyschromatopsia, and a central scotoma in one or both eyes may also occur. A relative afferent pupillary defect will be noted when the visual field loss in the two eyes is asymmetric. Optic disk pallor may occur when impairment has been long-standing.

A compressive lesion—pituitary tumor, craniopharyngioma, meningioma, aneurysm, mucocele—is the usual cause of a chiasmal syndrome. A glioma may occur in children, particularly those with neurofibromatosis. Demyelination and trauma are rare causes.

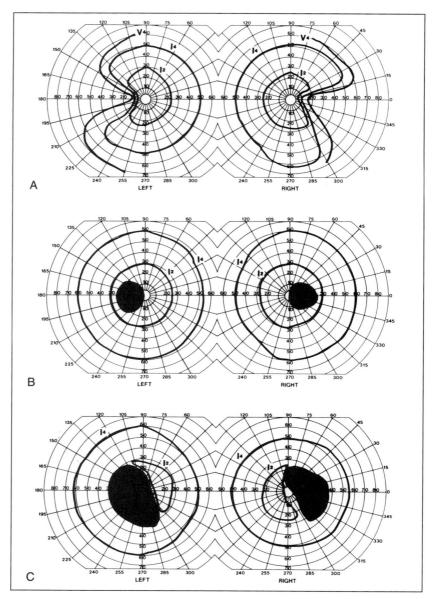

Fig. 1-14.
Nonchiasmal causes of bitemporal visual field defects. Note that the defects do not extend to or respect the vertical meridian in any of these cases. A. Congenitally tilted optic disks. B. Enlarged blind spots from papilledema. C. Sectoral retinitis pigmentosa.

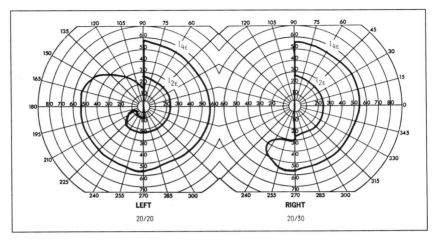

Fig. 1-15.
Optic tract syndrome. Compression of right optic tract by a craniopharyngioma. Note incongruity of visual field loss. (From C. H. Smith and R. W. Beck. The neuro-ophthalmic examination. Neurol. Clin. *1:807, 1983. Reprinted with permission from W. B. Saunders Co.)*

Bitemporal visual field loss does not always indicate a chiasmal lesion. Other causes include tilted optic disks, nasal sector retinitis pigmentosa, papilledema with markedly enlarged blind spots, bilateral cecocentral scotomas, and hysteria. In these entities, the visual field defects will not extend exactly to the vertical meridian as they will with a chiasmal lesion (Fig. 1-14).

OPTIC TRACT
Lesions of the visual system beyond the chiasm produce homonymous loss of visual field in the two eyes. Optic tract localization is supported by the presence of an incongruous homonymous hemianopia (Fig. 1-15). Decreased visual acuity, a relative afferent pupillary defect, and optic atrophy may occur with lesions of the optic tract but never with acquired lesions posterior to the tract, an important diagnostic point. Compressive lesions, in particular craniopharyngioma or pituitary tumor, are the usual causes of an optic tract syndrome.

GENICULOCALCARINE VISUAL SYSTEM
Lesions of the geniculocalcarine visual system produce a homonymous visual field defect, never reduce visual acuity when the lesion is unilateral, and never affect pupillary reaction or optic disk appearance. (The only exception to this is a congenital homonymous hemianopia in which a transsynaptic degeneration may result in optic atrophy.)

With a temporal lobe lesion, a homonymous superior visual defect may occur, whereas with a parietal lobe lesion, a homonymous hemianopia that is either complete or more dense inferiorly is possible (Fig. 1-16).

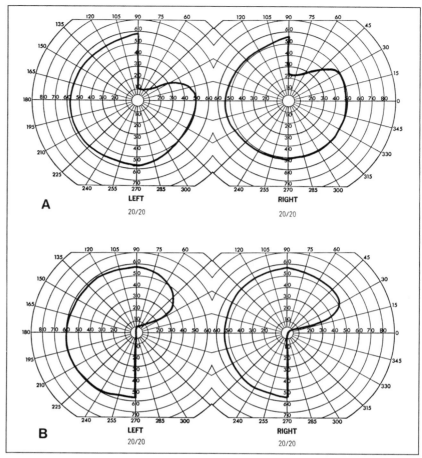

Fig. 1-16.
A. Left temporal lobe lesion producing slightly incongruous right superior quadran-
tanopsia. Note that the defect is slightly more extensive in the left eye than in the right
eye. B. Left parietal lobe lesion producing right homonymous hemianopia affecting
inferior field more than superior. (From C. H. Smith and R. W. Beck. The neuro-
ophthalmic examination. Neurol. Clin. 1:807, 1983. Reprinted with permission from
W. B. Saunders Co.)

An occipital lobe lesion is recognized by a homonymous hemianopia
that is exquisitely congruous. The macular representation (central 5 degrees of the visual field) or the temporal crescent (the most peripheral
30 degrees of the visual field), which is monocular, may be spared or
solely involved (Fig. 1-17).

Fig. 1-17.
Examples of visual field defects from occipital lobe lesions. A. A lesion of the left supe-
rior calcarine cortex producing a congruous right inferior quadrantanopsia. B. A le-
sion of the left posterior occipital cortex producing a congruous right homonymous
macular scotoma. C. Bilateral occipital lobe infarctions sparing the macular representa-
tion (posterior occipital cortex) on both sides. (continued on p. 26.)

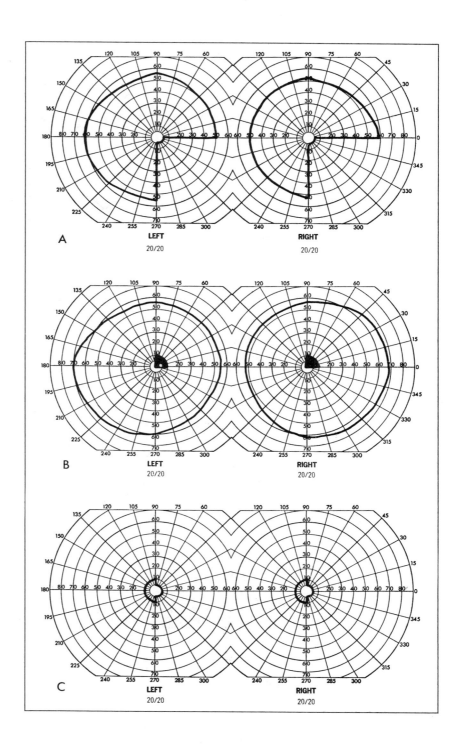

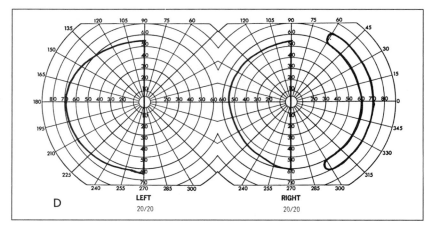

Fig. 1-17 (continued).
D. An infarction involving the entire left occipital lobe, except the anteriormost portion, producing a right homonymous hemianopia with sparing of the temporal crescent in the right eye. (From C. H. Smith and R. W. Beck. The neuro-ophthalmic examination. Neurol. Clin. 1:807, 1983. Reprinted with permission from W. B. Saunders Co.)

Temporal lobe lesions are usually the result of tumor, whereas parietal and occipital lesions are more often vascular.

Evaluation of the Oculomotor System

Impairment of ocular motility occurs with disorders of the extraocular muscles, neuromuscular junction, ocular motor nerves, brainstem nuclei, or supranuclear pathways. Examination of the ocular motor system should always consist of assessing the range of the excursion of each eye as well as both saccadic and pursuit eye movements.

Disorders of the ocular motor system often produce diplopia. In the evaluation for a cause it is important first to determine whether the diplopia is monocular or binocular. Monocular diplopia is usually due to a corneal, lens, macular, or refractive abnormality and only rarely has a neurologic basis.

When diplopia is binocular, certain questions should be asked of the patient about the onset and subsequent status of the diplopia. Often this information will be helpful in determining a diagnosis. The typical history of diplopia in various disorders is described in the box on page 27. It is also useful to ask the patient whether diplopia is worse in any position of gaze or at distance or near. The worst position of gaze will represent the field of action of a paretic muscle or be opposite the field of action of a restricted muscle. Diplopia worse in the distance suggests lateral rectus weakness, whereas diplopia worse at near suggests medial rectus weakness or convergence insufficiency.

On examining the patient with diplopia, one should observe the movement of the eyes into the cardinal positions of gaze before measuring the ocular deviation with prisms. If movement of an eye into a cer-

Disorder	Typical History
Ischemic nerve palsy	Sudden, nonprogressive
Graves' disease	Intermittent at onset; may become constant; worse on awakening in the morning
Myasthenia gravis	Intermittent at onset; may become constant; varies during the day; particularly worse later in day when patient is fatigued
Compressive lesions	Progressive worsening

tain direction is limited, this will provide a clue to diagnosis and obviate the need for complicated multipositional prism measurements. If the cause of diplopia is not obvious after observing the excursions of the eyes, then the deviation of the eyes in the cardinal positions of gaze must be measured. This can be done by cross-cover testing, with a red lens, or by other techniques. For vertical deviations, the Bielschowsky three-step test may be helpful for diagnosis (see Vertical Deviations, later in this chapter).

In certain circumstances other tests are of value:

1. Oculocephalics (doll's eyes), Bell's phenomenon, and calorics are useful in assessing whether an ophthalmoplegia is supranuclear.
2. Forced duction testing should be done when there is a possibility that a limitation in motility is due to a restrictive process.
3. A Tensilon test should be performed when myasthenia gravis is considered as a potential diagnosis.
4. Fusional amplitudes should be measured when diplopia may be due to the breakdown of a long-standing deviation. Supranormal amplitudes suggest a congenital problem.
5. Measurement of a cyclodeviation may be of value in determining the cause of vertical diplopia.
6. Review of old photographs may demonstrate a head tilt or face turn that would indicate that the deviation is long-standing.
7. Other portions of the ophthalmic evaluation that should be stressed include evaluation of the eyelids (lid retraction would suggest thyroid ophthalmopathy; ptosis might indicate myasthenia gravis), exophthalmometry and globe retropulsion, and the pupillary examination.

Causes of Diplopia

Heterophoria. Breakdown of a preexisting heterophoria should be considered particularly when there is a history of intermittence of the diplopia with the findings of a full range of eye movements and a concomitant deviation. Fusional amplitudes may be larger than normal.

Acquired Horizontal Deviations. An exotropia could be produced by medial rectus weakness or lateral rectus restriction. Medial rectus weakness may be produced by an internuclear ophthalmoplegia (lesion in the medial longitudinal fasciculus in the brainstem), myasthenia gravis, or a third nerve palsy (in which case there should be other signs of third nerve involvement). Lateral rectus restriction is an uncommon manifestation of Graves' ophthalmopathy.

There are numerous causes of abduction deficits producing esotropia. A sixth nerve palsy is the most common cause of isolated lateral rectus weakness. Such a palsy produces an esotropia that is greatest in the field of action of the weak lateral rectus and is greater at distance than near. Other disorders that can produce an abduction deficit include myasthenia gravis, medial rectus restriction from thyroid ophthalmopathy or orbital trauma, Duane's retraction syndrome, convergence spasm, and cross-fixation with a congenital esotropia.

Vertical Deviations. With vertical deviations it is particularly important to assess the motility before measuring the ocular deviation in various positions of gaze. Limitation of upgaze, either unilateral or bilateral, is a common cause of a hypertropia (see Chapter 22). Differential diagnosis would include inferior rectus restriction from thyroid ophthalmopathy or a blowout fracture, myasthenia gravis, third nerve (superior division) palsy, Brown's syndrome, skew deviation, supranuclear or nuclear impairment (Parinaud's syndrome as an example), and congenital double elevator palsy. In assessing the cause of impaired upgaze it is important to look for lid signs of thyroid ophthalmopathy or myasthenia gravis, perform oculocephalics to rule out a supranuclear lesion, perform forced ductions, and if the diagnosis is in doubt, do a Tensilon test.

Impaired downgaze is less frequently encountered but could be the result of a third nerve palsy, superior rectus restriction, myasthenia gravis, skew deviation, or other brainstem or supranuclear disorders.

When a diagnosis for vertical diplopia cannot be reached by the motility examination alone, the Bielschowsky three-step test is invaluable. The steps to follow are outlined in Fig. 1-18.

Listed in the box below is each muscle that when weak will produce a specified deviation.

Step 1	Step 2 Right gaze	Left gaze	Step 3 Right tilt	Left tilt
Right hypertropia				
RSO		RSO	RSO	
RIR	RIR			RIR
LIO	LIO		LIO	
LSR		LSR		LSR
Left hypertropia				
LSO	LSO			LSO
LIR		LIR	LIR	
RIO		RIO		RIO
RSR	RSR		RSR	

For each abbreviation, the first letter refers to right or left. The remainder of the abbreviation is as follows: SO = superior oblique; IO = inferior oblique; SR = superior rectus; IR = inferior rectus.

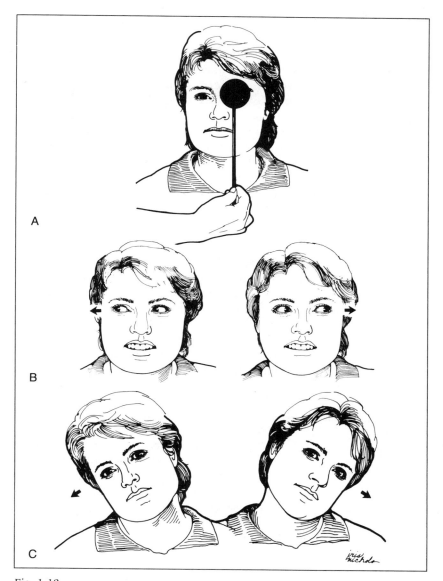

Fig. 1-18.

Demonstration of the Bielschowsky three-step test. A. Step 1. *Determine whether there is a right or left hypertropia in the primary position. The four muscles that when weak will produce a right hypertropia and the four that will produce a left hypertropia are listed in the table on p. 28.* B. Step 2. *Determine whether the deviation is greater in right or left gaze. With a right hypertropia the deviation will be greater in right gaze with two of the muscles and on left gaze with two muscles. The same is true for the four muscles producing a left hypertropia.* C. Step 3. *Determine whether the deviation is greater on right or left head tilt. With head tilt to the right, the intorters of the right eye (right superior oblique and right superior rectus) and the extorters of the left eye (left inferior oblique, left inferior rectus) will be activated, while the other four muscles will be inhibited. The reverse is true on head tilt to the left. If one of the activated muscles is weak, the vertical deviation will be greater on head tilt to that side. Combining the three steps will generally point to one muscle as being weak.*

Other tests that may be useful include measurement of the cyclodeviation using two Maddox rods and measurement of vertical fusional amplitudes using prisms. The former is particularly useful in diagnosing a superior oblique palsy since an excyclodeviation will usually be present, while the latter is helpful when a congenital motility disorder is being considered. Since the normal vertical fusional amplitude is only about 2.5 prism diopters, amplitudes that greatly exceed this suggest a long-standing or congenital problem.

The three-step test is most helpful in diagnosing a fourth nerve palsy. With a right fourth nerve palsy there is a right hypertropia that is greater on left gaze and right head tilt. The reverse is true with a left fourth nerve palsy. With bilateral palsies, the deviation in the primary position may be small and there is right hypertropia on left gaze and right head tilt and a left hypertropia on right gaze and left head tilt.

SUMMARY OF IMPORTANT POINTS
1. Remember to observe the motility pattern carefully before measuring the ocular deviation in the cardinal positions or performing a three-step test.
2. Examine the eyelids and orbits, because they may have signs that are helpful in diagnosis.
3. After observing the ocular motility and measuring the deviation in the cardinal positions when indicated, first decide whether the motility pattern can be explained by involvement of the third, fourth, or sixth cranial nerve. If not, then consider other disorders.
4. With medial rectus weakness, consider internuclear ophthalmoplegia or myasthenia.
5. With lateral rectus weakness, consider sixth nerve palsy but remember the other causes of abduction deficits.
6. Consider myasthenia gravis and thyroid ophthalmopathy, particularly when a deviation is not following a neurogenic pattern. These disorders can produce a wide variety of ocular deviations.

Nystagmus

Nystagmus refers to a rhythmic oscillation of the eyes. When a patient with nystagmus is examined, the eyes should be observed first in the primary position and then in the different positions of gaze and convergence. It should be noted whether (1) there is a specific direction for a fast phase or whether the nystagmus appears pendular, (2) the nystagmus is similar in the two eyes, (3) a null point exists, and (4) there is a latent component (increase in nystagmus when one eye is covered). The examiner must look carefully for a torsional component as it can easily be missed and must keep in mind the possibility of a periodic alternating nystagmus. When nystagmus is of low amplitude, it may be easier to detect by viewing the fundus with a direct ophthalmoscope than with the naked eye.

Congenital nystagmus is a benign condition present from birth. It may appear as pendular or jerk, typically appears similar in the two eyes, is horizontal, and decreases with convergence. An inverted optokinetic nystagmus response may be present. Latent nystagmus may accompany congenital nystagmus or an esotropia.

There are many forms of acquired nystagmus. A detailed discussion is beyond the scope of this book, but some of the more common forms with localizing value are listed in Table 1-4.

Pupils

The pupillary examination provides an objective assessment of the integrity of the visual system from the retina through the optic tract, as well as an indication of the function of the efferent parasympathetic and sympathetic systems (Fig. 1-19). The testing for a relative afferent pupillary defect is described earlier in this chapter.

Anisocoria is evaluated by recording pupil size under both bright and dim illumination. Figure 1-20 provides a schematic approach to the examination of a patient with anisocoria, and Table 1-5 reviews the common eyedrops that are useful in diagnosis. When the anisocoria is greater in darkness than in light, a sympathetic paresis is present and the miotic pupil is the abnormal one. When anisocoria is greater in light than in darkness, the parasympathetic system is impaired and it is the larger pupil that is abnormal. If the difference in pupil size is the same under both conditions, essential anisocoria, which is of no neurologic importance, is probably present. In about 20 percent of the population there is a difference in pupil size of at least 1 mm.

Table 1-4. Types of nystagmus and their neurologic localization

Type	Localization
Downbeat	Craniocervical junction
Periodic alternating	Craniocervical junction
Gaze-evoked	Vestibular, cerebellum
Upbeat	Cerebellum, medulla
Seesaw	Diencephalon, mesencephalon
Torsional	Central vestibular
Convergence-retraction	Dorsal midbrain
Rebound	Cerebellum

Table 1-5. Pharmacologic testing

Drug	Entity	Abnormal pupil	Normal pupil
Cocaine hydrochloride 4–10%	Horner's	Less dilation	Dilation
Pilocarpine ⅛–1/16%	Adie's	Constriction	Less constriction
Pilocarpine 1%	Pharmacologic	No constriction	Constriction

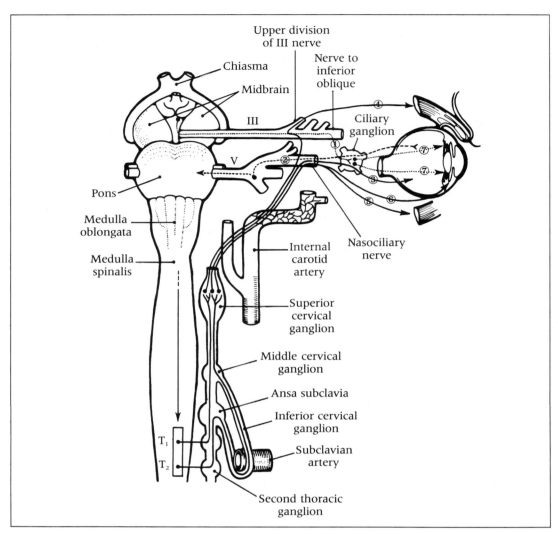

Fig. 1-19.
Anatomy of the parasympathetic and sympathetic pupillary pathways. 1. Parasympathetic (motor) root. 2. Sensory root. 3. Sympathetic (vasomotor) root. 4. Sympathetic nerve to Müller's muscle in levator palpebrae superioris. 5. Sympathetic nerve to Müller's muscle. 6. Sympathetic nerve to dilator pupillae. 7. Parasympathetic nerve to ciliary muscle and sphincter pupillae. Key: ——— = sympathetic; . . . = parasympathetic; --- = sensory.

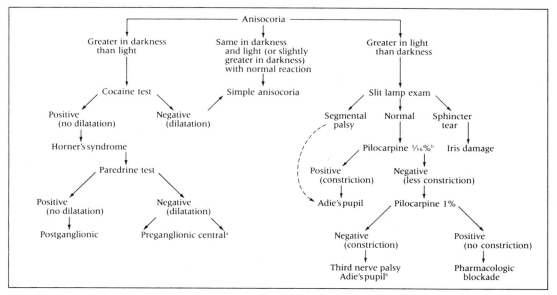

Fig. 1-20.

Approach to the patient with anisocoria. (Adapted from H. S. Thompson and S. F. J. Pilley. Unequal pupils. A flow chart for sorting out the anisocorias. Surv. Ophthalmol. *21:45, 1976. With permission.)*

[a] *There is no good drug test to separate a preganglionic from a central lesion.*

[b] *In approximately 20 percent of cases of Adie's pupil, pilocarpine 1/16% does not constrict the pupil.*

A sympathetic paresis represents Horner's syndrome, whereas parasympathetic impairment could be due to a third nerve palsy, Adie's syndrome, pharmacologic blockade, or a damaged iris sphincter.

Pupillary constriction may occur not only from stimulation of the eyes with light but also as part of the near triad (accommodation, convergence, pupillary constriction). Some conditions may impair the light response without affecting the near response (light-near dissociation): Parinaud's (dorsal midbrain) syndrome, neurosyphilis, diabetes mellitus, Adie's pupil, aberrant third nerve regeneration, and bilateral severe optic neuropathy.

References

1. Glaser, J. S., et al. The photostress recovery test in the clinical assessment of visual function. *Am. J. Ophthalmol.* 83:255, 1977.
2. Levatin, P. Pupillary escape in disease of the retina or optic nerve. *Arch. Ophthalmol.* 62:768, 1959.
3. Thompson, H. S. Pupillary signs in the diagnosis of optic nerve disease. *Trans. Ophthalmol. Soc. U.K.* 96:377, 1976.
4. Trobe, J. D., et al. An evaluation of the accuracy of community-based perimetry. *Am. J. Ophthalmol.* 90:654, 1980.

2

Optic Neuritis

A 21-year-old woman noted blurred vision in the right eye associated with a dull ache around the eye, which worsened on eye movement. Visual loss had progressed over the 5-day period before her examination. Her history was unremarkable.

Neuro-Ophthalmic Examination

	OD	OS
Visual acuity	20/400	20/20
Color plates correct	Missed control	10 of 10
Pupils	Relative afferent pupillary defect	
Motility, lids, orbits	Normal	Normal
Fundi	Normal	Normal

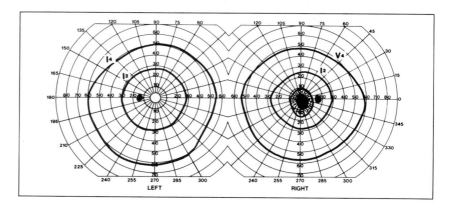

Results of a neurologic examination were normal.

Summary
A 21-year-old woman presented with acute monocular visual loss and on examination was found to have decreased visual acuity in the right eye with a central scotoma, a relative afferent pupillary defect, and a normal-appearing optic disk.

34

Differential Diagnosis

An acute monocular retrobulbar optic neuropathy in this age group is most probably due to optic neuritis. Other possible causes include sinus disease (mucocele), vasculitis, and infiltration of the nerve with a carcinomatous, lymphoreticular, or granulomatous process. A compressive lesion would be unusual because of the rapidity of visual loss. Meningiomas and gliomas generally produce gradual visual loss over weeks to months, but craniopharyngiomas occasionally produce fairly rapid loss. Pituitary apoplexy is a remote possibility, but chiasmal involvement is more likely than optic nerve. Other unlikely possibilities include nutritional and toxic processes, which almost always affect both eyes to some degree, and Leber's hereditary optic neuropathy, which could present in this manner but would be unusual in a female.

Clinical Diagnosis: Optic Neuritis

There are a number of possible causes of optic neuritis, but in many cases a specific cause cannot be discerned. The pathogenesis of optic neuritis is generally considered to be immune-mediated demyelination of the optic nerve. Although only 20 to 50 percent of patients with optic neuritis are ultimately found to have multiple sclerosis (MS), similarities between the two in incidence, cerebrospinal fluid (CSF) findings, magnetic resonance imaging (MRI) abnormalities, histocompatibility data, family history, and various clinical features suggest that optic neuritis may be a *forme fruste* of multiple sclerosis. In a small percentage of cases, primary demyelination is not the cause, and another cause such as syphilis, sarcoidosis, or a viral or postviral syndrome is identified. A viral or postviral syndrome is a common cause in children (see Chapter 3).

The diagnosis of optic neuritis rests on clinical grounds. Patients developing idiopathic or MS-related optic neuritis are usually between the ages of 15 and 45 years. Visual loss is acute but may progress for 7 to 10 days. Progression for a longer time is possible but should make the clinician suspicious of an alternative cause. Pain usually exacerbated by eye movement may precede or coincide with visual loss. It generally lasts less than 2 weeks. Visual acuity is reduced in most cases but varies from a mild reduction to severe loss (no light perception possible). Color vision is impaired in almost all cases and is often impaired out of proportion to acuity (see Chapter 1). The typical visual field defect is a central scotoma, although in about 10 percent of cases central fixation is spared and another type of defect is present. A relative afferent pupillary defect will be detectable in almost all unilateral cases. If such a defect is not present, a preexisting optic neuropathy in the fellow eye should be suspected. This is not uncommon in multiple sclerosis, in which subclinical demyelination may occur without visual symptoms. The optic disk may appear normal (retrobulbar neuritis) or swollen (papillitis) in optic neuritis, and clinical features are similar regardless. In a small percentage of cases, optic neuritis will simultaneously affect both eyes.

Regardless of the degree of impairment of vision, visual function in most cases of optic neuritis begins improving one to several weeks after the onset. Approximately 85 percent of patients will have final visual acuity of 20/40 or better. Even with good recovery of acuity, however, there are frequently residual deficits in color vision, contrast sensitivity, light brightness sense, and stereopsis that may be disabling. A relative afferent pupillary defect and optic disk pallor are usually still detectable, and the visually evoked potential latency almost always remains prolonged. The patient may complain of loss of vision with exercise (Uhthoff's phenomenon).

Additional Testing

If the patient's clinical course is typical for optic neuritis, further testing need not be extensive. An antinuclear antibody (ANA) determination should be considered, particularly if there are any symptoms of collagen vascular disease, and sinus x-rays may be indicated if the history suggests previous sinus disease. We generally do not recommend a computed tomography (CT) scan, MRI scan, lumbar puncture, or evoked potentials when the course is typical, unless the patient requests that all tests that might further define a diagnosis of multiple sclerosis be performed. However, CSF and MRI abnormalities do not necessarily predict whether the patient will develop clinical signs of MS. CSF changes in optic neuritis are similar to those in MS in general. Elevations in immunoglobulin G (IgG) and oligoclonal banding have been reported in 24 to 55 percent of optic neuritis patients. MRI scans of the brain are abnormal in about 60 percent. CT may demonstrate enlargement of the nerves.

If the course becomes atypical—visual loss progresses for more than 10 days, pain persists, or other symptoms develop—a CT or MRI scan and a lumbar puncture may be in order in an attempt to make a more definitive diagnosis.

Treatment

Therapy in optic neuritis remains controversial. Corticosteroids are often prescribed, but evidence of their efficacy is lacking. No clinical study has considered a sufficient number of patients to determine whether treatment is of value. It has been our clinical impression that corticosteroids in some patients dramatically speed recovery but whether the ultimate outcome would be different is unknown. A reasonable approach is to discuss the controversy of treatment and the short-term side effects of corticosteroids with the patient and decide with him or her on whether therapy should be given. If the patient has a contraindication to corticosteroids, such as diabetes mellitus, gastric ulcers, or exposure to tuberculosis, it is prudent to not treat. Specific circumstances in which we generally advocate treatment include (1) cases in which the patient has only one eye or in which the fellow eye has poor vision, (2) a previous episode of optic neuritis treated with corticosteroids in which there was good recovery, and (3) disabling or persistent periocular pain. When oral corticosteroids are prescribed, initial doses range from 60 to 100 mg of prednisone. Two to three weeks of therapy should be the maximum in most patients. High-dose intravenous methylprednisolone (1 gm/day) has been used in acute exacerbations of multiple sclerosis with good results. Although it has not been extensively studied in optic neuritis, preliminary results indicate that with this therapy a very rapid recovery of vision is possible.

Relationship to Multiple Sclerosis

How much the patient with optic neuritis should be told about multiple sclerosis is a question frequently posed by the clinician. The answer must be individualized for each patient. It must be remembered that multiple sclerosis is a spectrum of disease in which a downhill, disabling course is not the fate of all patients. Isolated optic neuritis may remain at one end of the spectrum. If the physician decides to discuss the issue with the patient, the physician should feel obligated to discuss it in detail, indicating to the patient exactly what a diagnosis of MS means and not just mentioning the diagnosis in passing. Often the patient will have heard about the association between MS and optic neuritis and will ask the physician about it. If not, it is reasonable not to even discuss the issue with the patient who has no other neurologic symptoms or signs.

Recurrence

Optic neuritis recurs in approximately 20 percent of cases. With each succeeding episode in an eye, the chances for visual recovery decrease.

Management and Course of the Case

Since on presentation the case appeared typical for optic neuritis, additional testing consisted only of an ANA blood test, which had normal results. The pros and cons of corticosteroid therapy were discussed with the patient and a decision was made to not treat her. The issue of multiple sclerosis was not raised. The patient was examined after 2 weeks, at which time visual acuity and the visual field were unchanged. One month later visual acuity had improved to 20/60. Three and six months later visual acuity was 20/20 and perimetric results were normal. She still had a relative afferent pupillary defect and had developed moderate optic disk pallor.

Papillitis

A 22-year-old man who developed sudden visual loss in the left eye was found to have visual acuity of 20/200, a left relative afferent pupillary defect, a central scotoma in the visual field, and a swollen left optic disk (see Plate 1). A diagnosis of optic neuritis (papillitis) was made.

Optic neuritis may occur with a normal or swollen disk. In the former case it is called retrobulbar neuritis, in the latter, papillitis. Clinical features of the two are similar.

Optic Neuritis Mimic: Sphenoidal Mucocele

A 30-year-old woman with acute visual loss in the left eye was found on examination 1 week later to have visual acuity of 20/40, a left relative afferent pupillary defect, a central scotoma in the visual field, and a normal funduscopic appearance. A diagnosis of optic neuritis was made; no treatment was instituted.

On examination 2 weeks later, visual acuity had decreased in the left eye to 20/200, and the visual field was worse. The optic disk again appeared normal. The right eye remained normal.

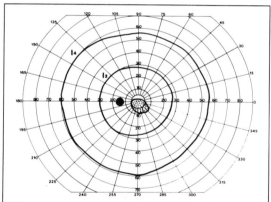

Initial field.   Field after 2 weeks.

The progression of visual loss for more than 1 week was atypical for optic neuritis, and a CT scan was performed. It demonstrated a sphenoidal mucocele (see photo on page 39).

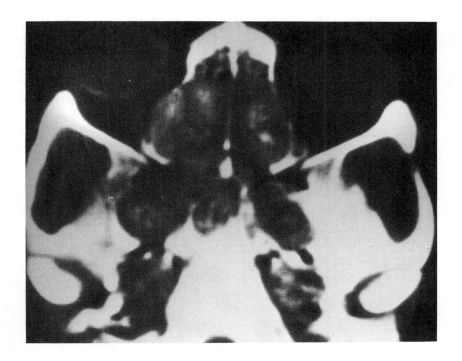

Optic Neuritis Mimic: Craniopharyngioma

A 36-year-old woman noted visual loss in the left eye while reading. Visual acuity was 20/20 in the right eye and 20/30 in the left eye, she missed 6 of 11 color plates with the left eye, and a left relative afferent pupillary defect was present. The fundus appeared normal. Her visual field is shown below.

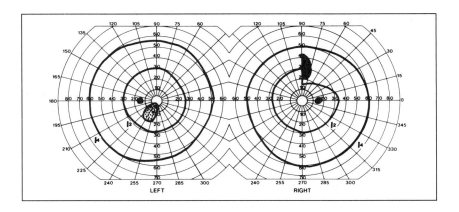

Although the history was consistent with optic neuritis, the presence of a temporal visual field defect in the right eye localized the process to the posterior optic nerve and was most suggestive of a compressive lesion. A CT scan was interpreted as normal. Because a compressive lesion remained a strong possibility, a metrizamide CT scan was performed (metrizamide dye was injected through a lumbar puncture before computed tomography) and demonstrated a cystic mass with flecks of calcium in the suprasellar cistern (see below).

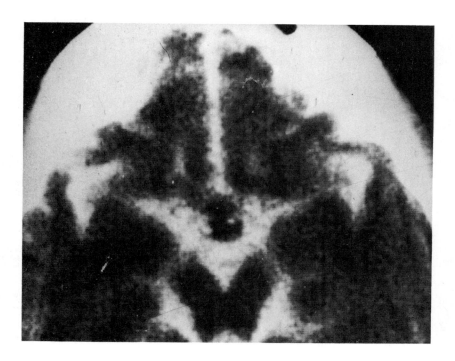

At surgery a craniopharyngioma was removed. Today a magnetic resonance imaging scan, if available, would be preferable to a metrizamide CT scan and would probably provide the diagnosis.

This case demonstrates the importance of carefully evaluating the visual field in the fellow eye in cases thought to be unilateral optic neuritis. Although visual loss was reported as acute, it may have been present for some time and was just discovered suddenly by the patient. This case also stresses the importance of a thorough investigation for a compressive lesion when the disease can be localized to the posterior optic nerve or chiasm.

Bibliography

Burde, R. M., et al. Central visual dysfunction with disc swelling. *Surv. Oph-thalmol.* 26:43, 1981.

Cohen, M. M., Lessell, S., and Wolf, P. A. A prospective study of the risk of developing multiple sclerosis in uncomplicated optic neuritis. *Neurology* 29: 208, 1979.

Ebers, G. C. Optic neuritis and multiple sclerosis. *Arch. Neurol.* 42:702, 1985.

Fleishman, J. A., and Beck, R. W. Visual function after resolution of optic neuritis. *Ophthalmology* (in press).

Nikoskelainen, E., Frey, H., and Salmi, A. Prognosis of optic neuritis with special reference to cerebrospinal fluid immunoglobulins and measles virus antibodies. *Ann. Neurol.* 9:545, 1981.

Ormerod, I. E. C., et al. Disseminated lesions at presentation in patients with optic neuritis. *J. Neurol. Neurosurg. Psychiatry* 49:124, 1986.

Perkin, G. D., and Rose, F. C. *Optic Neuritis and Its Differential Diagnosis.* Oxford, England: Oxford University Press, 1979.

Sergott, R. C., et al. Optic nerve demyelination induced by human serum: Patients with multiple sclerosis or optic neuritis and normal subjects. *Neurology* 35:1438, 1985.

3

Optic Neuritis in a Child

A 9-year-old girl rapidly lost vision in first the right and then the left eye over a 4-day period. She had a dull bifrontal headache. Two weeks earlier she had experienced an upper respiratory infection with a low-grade fever for several days.

Neuro-Ophthalmic Examination

	OD	OS
Visual acuity	Light perception	Finger counting
Pupils	Sluggish	Sluggish
Motility, lids, orbits	Normal	Normal
Fundi (see Plate 2)	Swollen optic disk	Swollen optic disk

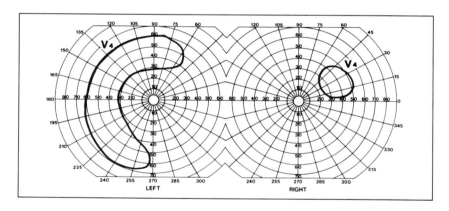

Results of a neurologic examination were normal.

Summary
A 9-year-old girl developed severe bilateral visual loss associated with marked loss of visual field and optic disk edema in both eyes.

Differential Diagnosis

Acute bilateral visual loss in a child probably results from optic neuritis. A postviral (parainfectious) syndrome is the most common cause. Multiple sclerosis is less likely. Other possible causes are vasculitis, sarcoidosis, syphilis, infiltration with a carcinomatous or lymphomatous process, sinusitis, bacterial meningitis, and a toxin. Heavy metal poisoning and various drugs can affect the optic nerves, but without a history of ingestion and with evidence of optic disk edema, these would be unlikely. A compressive lesion would be extremely unlikely in view of the optic disk edema and nonchiasmal pattern of visual field loss. Increased intracranial pressure could produce the funduscopic picture but would not be expected to produce the visual loss acutely. Leber's optic neuropathy (see Chapter 11) can rapidly produce severe visual loss in both eyes but would be unusual at this age and in a female.

Differential diagnosis would be similar in an adult with bilateral optic disk edema and acute visual loss except that multiple sclerosis might be more likely than a postviral syndrome. In patients older than 60, giant cell arteritis would be a likely possibility.

Clinical Diagnosis: Parainfectious (Postviral) Optic Neuritis

Parainfectious optic neuritis typically follows the onset of a viral infection by 1 to 3 weeks. It has been associated with rubeola, rubella, mumps, varicella, herpes zoster, infectious mononucleosis, enterovirus, and other viruses, and has occurred as a postvaccination phenomenon. The optic neuritis is felt to be due to an immunologic process that produces demyelination of the optic nerve. An immune-mediated meningoencephalitis is frequently associated and may be asymptomatic.

The optic neuritis may be unilateral but more commonly is bilateral. Visual loss is generally severe. The optic disks may appear normal or swollen. Fortunately visual recovery is usually excellent.

Additional Testing

Computed tomography (CT) is unlikely to provide useful information, but because of the usual severity and bilaterality of visual loss, the clinician in most cases will order the scan. Optic nerve enlargement should not concern the clinician since this can occur with optic neuritis. The scan will be useful to evaluate for sinus disease.

A lumbar puncture is frequently helpful in diagnosis. In many cases of parainfectious optic neuritis there will be a pleocytosis with a lymphocytic predominance and an elevation in the cerebrospinal fluid protein.

If the cerebrospinal fluid examination does not support a parainfectious diagnosis, serologic tests for collagen vascular disease should be performed.

Treatment

Although the natural history of visual loss may be recovery without treatment, corticosteroid therapy is advised in most patients, particularly when involvement is bilateral. Recovery of vision often begins within several days after therapy commences and is frequently complete within 1 month. Steroids are begun with prednisone in a dosage of 1 to 2 mg per kg for 2 weeks and then tapered over the succeeding month. In a small percentage of cases visual loss will recur as the steroids are tapered, necessitating an increase in the dosage and a slower taper.

Management and Course of the Case

A CT scan showed mild diffuse enlargement of the optic nerves but was otherwise normal. On lumbar puncture the opening pressure was 180 mm of water. The cerebrospinal fluid contained 180 lymphocytes and had a protein level of 95 mg/dl and a glucose level of 70 mg/dl.

The patient was placed on a regimen of 40 mg of prednisone per day. Visual recovery began 3 days later, and over a 1-month period visual acuity returned to 20/20 in each eye.

Neuroretinitis

A 6-year-old boy developed visual loss in the right eye. Visual acuity was finger counting, and the right optic disk was swollen with retinal exudates (see Plate 3). Toxoplasmosis and *Toxocara* titers were negative. A diagnosis of optic neuritis (neuroretinitis) was made, with the cause presumed to be postviral. He was treated with prednisone and recovered visual acuity of 20/20.

Neuroretinitis is a form of optic neuritis in which in addition to a swollen optic disk there is retinal exudation, which may take the form of a macular star. The prominence of the macular exudates led to the coining of the name *Leber's stellate maculopathy* for this condition. This entity is distinct from demyelinative optic neuritis. Neuroretinitis is almost never associated with multiple sclerosis. The cause is unknown in most cases but is often presumed to be postviral. Syphilis, histoplasmosis, cat-scratch fever, and leptospirosis have also been associated with this condition.

Bibliography

Dreyer, R. F., et al. Leber's idiopathic stellate neuroretinitis. *Arch. Ophthalmol.* 102:1140, 1984.

Frey, T. Optic neuritis in children: Infectious mononucleosis as an etiology. *Doc. Ophthalmol.* 34:183, 1973.

Kazarian, E. L., and Gager, W. E. Optic neuritis complicating measles, mumps, and rubella vaccination. *Am. J. Ophthalmol.* 86:544, 1978.

Maitland, C. G., and Miller, N. R. Neuroretinitis. *Arch. Ophthalmol.* 102:1146, 1984.

Parkin, P. J., Hierons, R., and McDonald, W. I. Bilateral optic neuritis: A long term follow-up. *Brain* 107:951, 1984.

Perry, H. D., et al. Reversible blindness in optic neuritis associated with influenza vaccination. *Ann. Ophthalmol.* 11:545, 1979.

Selbst, R. G., et al. Parainfectious optic neuritis: Report and review following varicella. *Arch. Neurol.* 40:347, 1983.

Silverstein, A. Papilledema and acute viral infections of the brain. *Mt. Sinai J. Med. (N.Y.)* 41:435, 1974.

4

Anterior Ischemic Optic Neuropathy

A 52-year-old man awoke with visual loss in the right eye. He had no pain, other symptoms, or preceding visual disturbances. His medical history was remarkable only for 5 years of essential hypertension, which was well controlled with a thiazide diuretic. The visual deficit had remained unchanged for the 1 week before examination.

Neuro-Ophthalmic Examination

	OD	OS
Visual acuity	20/30	20/20
Color plates correct	8 of 10	10 of 10
Pupils	Relative afferent pupillary defect	
Motility, lids, orbits	Normal	Normal
Fundi	Swollen optic disk (see Plate 4)	Normal

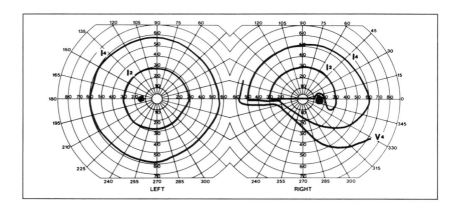

Summary

A 52-year-old man with sudden nonprogressive monocular visual loss was found on examination to have in the right eye visual acuity of 20/30, a relative afferent pupillary defect, an inferior altitudinal visual field defect, and a swollen optic disk.

Differential Diagnosis

Unilateral optic disk edema can occur with anterior ischemic optic neuropathy (AION), optic neuritis, orbital compressive lesions, central retinal vein occlusion, and optic nerve infiltration with a carcinomatous, granulomatous, or lymphoreticular process. Based on the patient's age, rapidity of onset, pattern of visual field loss, and optic disk appearance, anterior ischemic optic neuropathy is the most likely cause. Optic neuritis generally occurs at a younger age, and a central scotoma would be a more typical visual field defect. A central retinal vein occlusion occasionally can produce disk swelling with minimal retinal changes, but there is not usually visual field loss except for an enlarged blind spot. Orbital masses and infiltrative disorders generally produce progressive visual loss, and other clues to the diagnosis are usually present in the history or on examination.

Clinical Diagnosis: Anterior Ischemic Optic Neuropathy

Anterior ischemic optic neuropathy is characterized by acute visual loss, optic disk edema, and a visual field defect usually in a nerve fiber bundle distribution. Most cases of AION either are due to giant cell arteritis or, more commonly, are of unknown causation (and are referred to as idiopathic, nonarteritic, or atherosclerotic). Differentiation of the two forms is imperative since corticosteroid therapy will be of value for the arteritic but not the nonarteritic cases. The distinction can usually be made based on the history, clinical features, erythrocyte sedimentation rate (ESR), and in some cases a temporal artery biopsy. The clinical profile in arteritic AION is described in Chapter 5. Table 4-1 summarizes some of the differentiating features.

The usual patient developing nonarteritic AION is between 45 and 65 years old. Although there is an increased incidence of hypertension and diabetes mellitus, patients developing this condition are generally in good health without serious systemic complications of vascular disease.

Table 4-1. Features differentiating arteritic from nonarteritic anterior ischemic optic neuropathy (AION)

Characteristic	Arteritic AION	Nonarteritic AION
Age	Usually older than 60	Usually 45–65
Visual loss	Typically sudden and severe, may be progressive	Sudden, usually not as severe, nonprogressive
Ocular pain	May be present	Rare
Amaurosis fugax before AION	Occasional	Rare
Bilateral involvement	Common, within days–weeks	About 25%, within months–years
Optic disk appearance	Swollen, may be chalky white	Swollen; pale or hyperemic
Systemic symptoms	Usually present (see Chapter 5)	None
Physiologic cup size	Small or large	Usually small
Erythrocyte sedimentation rate	Usually elevated	Normal
Disk cupping in atrophic stage	Often marked	Mild or none

Visual loss is typically sudden and painless without preceding transient visual phenomena and is generally permanent. The deficit is usually at its worst from the onset, but in about 10 percent of cases may progress over a period of 2 to 3 weeks. Visual loss varies from mild to severe; in about one-third of cases visual acuity remains at or near 20/20. Visual field defects are generally in a nerve fiber bundle distribution (see Chapter 1) with the inferior field being affected three times more commonly than the superior. The visual field defect is generally permanent.

Recognition of optic disk edema in the acute phase is necessary for definitive diagnosis. The edema may be diffuse or sectoral, and the disk may appear hyperemic or pale. Peripapillary hemorrhages are common. In the usual patient, the edema resolves over a period of 1 to 2 months, and the involved portion of the disk becomes pale.

Once disk edema resolves, recurrences of AION in the same eye are rare. However, AION develops in the fellow eye in about 25 percent of cases, usually months to years after the initial involvement. When this occurs, a pseudo–Foster Kennedy syndrome (discussed later in this chapter) is produced.

Despite its common occurrence, the cause of nonarteritic AION is not well defined. It is likely to be multifactorial, with both atherosclerotic vascular changes and an underlying disk anomaly having roles. Several investigators have demonstrated that disks developing AION have a higher than expected incidence of a small or no physiologic cup. How this finding relates to the pathogenesis is unknown.

Additional Testing

The erythrocyte sedimentation rate should be obtained by the Westergren method if possible to aid in an evaluation for giant cell arteritis. Values greater than 40 mm per hour should be considered suspicious. If giant cell arteritis is a consideration, a temporal artery biopsy should be performed. With clinical features consistent with nonarteritic AION, a computed tomography scan and lumbar puncture are not indicated. They should be reserved for cases with atypical features in which other causes are a real consideration.

In regard to systemic vascular disease, approximately 40 percent of patients will have hypertension, and 10 percent diabetes. There is a slightly higher than expected incidence of cardiac and cerebrovascular disease but no increased risk of early death. Emboli do not play a major role in the pathogenesis, and the frequency of carotid artery disease is comparable on the involved and opposite sides. Thus it is advisable for patients with nonarteritic AION to have a general physical examination and an evaluation for hypertension and diabetes mellitus, but invasive or noninvasive carotid studies are not specifically indicated.

Treatment

No therapy is known to be of value. Corticosteroids have not proved to be efficacious and are generally not prescribed for this condition by most neuro-ophthalmologists. Antiplatelet therapy, such as with aspirin or dipyridamole (Persantine) should be considered as this may reduce the incidence of cardiac and cerebrovascular events in these patients.

Management and Course of the Case

The Westergren erythrocyte sedimentation rate was 5 mm per hour. A temporal artery biopsy was not performed. The patient was placed on a regimen of low-dose aspirin. On examination after 2 weeks, optic disk edema was still present and the visual field defect was unchanged. One month later the optic disk edema had resolved but again the visual field defect was unchanged. In 1 year of subsequent follow-up there was no change in his condition.

Pseudo–Foster Kennedy Syndrome

A 53-year-old man had acute visual loss in the left eye. One and one-half years earlier he had experienced sudden visual loss in the right eye associated with a swollen optic disk. Visual acuity was 20/20 in each eye. The right optic disk was pale and the left optic disk was swollen (see Plate 5). His visual field is shown below.

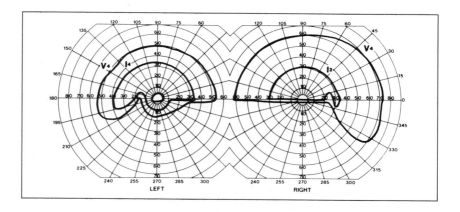

This patient experienced nonarteritic AION first in one and then the other eye. With second eye involvement a picture of disk edema in one eye and optic atrophy in the other eye is seen. This mimics Foster Kennedy syndrome, which results from an intracranial mass producing unilateral optic nerve compression (causing optic atrophy) and increased intracranial pressure. Consecutive AION in the two eyes occurs in about 25 percent of cases.

Arteritic AION with a Normal Sedimentation Rate

A 67-year-old woman who noted sudden painless visual loss in the right eye was found to have visual acuity of 20/50, a relative afferent pupillary defect, a mildly swollen optic disk, and a superior visual field defect in the right eye. On examination the left eye was completely normal. She had no symptoms of arteritis and a Westergren ESR was 28 mm per hour. A diagnosis of nonarteritic AION was made.

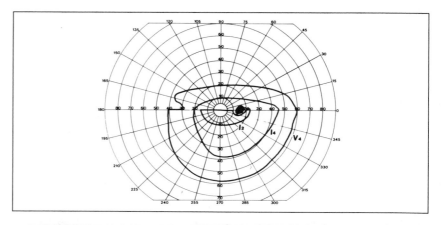

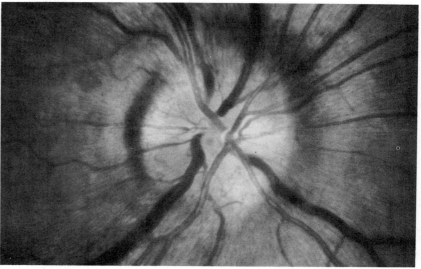

She returned 2 weeks later. Although she had not noted a change, visual acuity in the right eye was now reduced to finger counting and there was marked loss of visual field. The optic disk appearance had not changed, and the retina appeared normal. The left eye remained normal. She still felt well. A repeat ESR was 20 mm per hour.

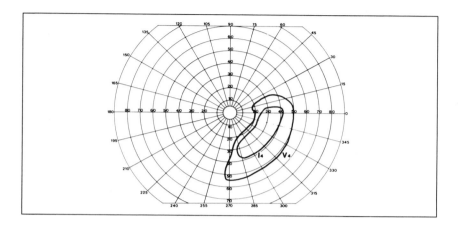

Because the progression of the visual loss was atypical for nonarteritic AION, a temporal artery biopsy was performed. The biopsy disclosed giant cell arteritis.

This case shows the possible occult nature of giant cell arteritis. This patient had no systemic symptoms of arteritis, and the ESR was normal. Progressive visual loss does occur in a small percentage of cases of nonarteritic AION, but it raises suspicion for giant cell arteritis and in this case was the only clue to the diagnosis. Giant cell arteritis should be considered whenever the clinical picture is atypical for nonarteritic AION, even if the ESR is normal.

Bibliography

Beck, R. W., et al. Anterior ischemic optic neuropathy: Recurrent episodes in the same eye. *Br. J. Ophthalmol.* 67:705, 1983.

Beck, R. W., et al. Optic disc cupping in anterior ischemic optic neuropathy: Comparison of arteritic and nonarteritic cases. *Ophthalmology* (in press).

Boghen, D. R., and Glaser, J. S. Ischemic optic neuropathy: The clinical profile and natural history. *Brain* 98:689, 1975.

Guyer, D. R., et al. The risk of cerebrovascular and cardiovascular disease in patients with anterior ischemic optic neuropathy. *Arch. Ophthalmol.* 103:1136, 1985.

Hayreh, S. S. Anterior ischemic optic neuropathy: I. Terminology and pathogenesis. II. Fundus on ophthalmoscopy and fluorescein angiography. III. Treatment, prophylaxis, and differential diagnosis. *Br. J. Ophthalmol.* 58:955, 1974.

Hayreh, S. S., and Chopdar, A. Occlusion of the posterior ciliary artery: V. Protective influence of simultaneous vortex vein occlusion. *Arch. Ophthalmol.* 100:1481, 1982.

Quigley, H. A., Miller, N. R., and Green, W. R. The pattern of optic nerve fiber loss in anterior ischemic optic neuropathy. *Am. J. Ophthalmol.* 100:769, 1985.

Repka, M. X., et al. Clinical profile and long-term implications of anterior ischemic optic neuropathy. *Am. J. Ophthalmol.* 96:478, 1983.

Shults, W. T. Ischemic optic neuropathy: Still the ophthalmologist's dilemma. *Ophthalmology* 91:1338, 1984.

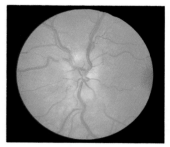

1. Papillitis OS in a 22-year-old man.

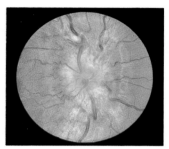

OD

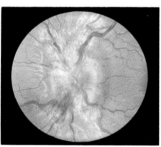

OS

2. Bilateral optic neuritis in a 9-year-old girl.

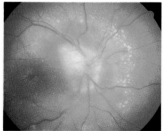

3. Neuroretinitis OD in a 6-year-old boy.

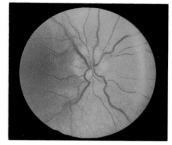

4. Swollen optic disk from anterior ischemic optic neuropathy in a 52-year-old man: OD.

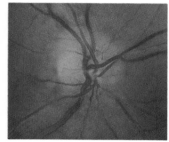

OD

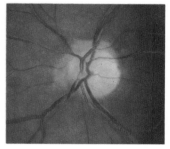

OS

5. Pseudo-Foster Kennedy syndrome with optic disk edema OD and optic atrophy OS in a 53-year-old man.

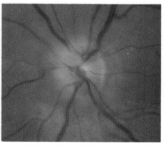

6. Pallid swelling of the left optic disk in a 72-year-old woman with giant cell arteritis.

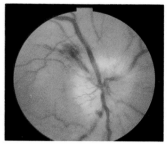

OD

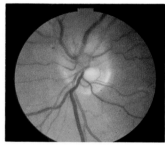

OS

7. Pallid swelling of the right disk and mild swelling of the superior left disk in a 69-year-old man with giant cell arteritis.

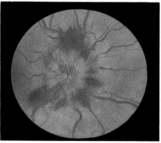

OD

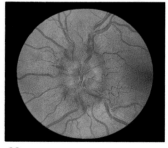

OS

8. Bilateral papilledema in a 21-year-old woman with pseudotumor cerebri.

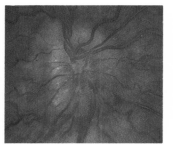

OD

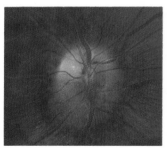

OS

9. Bilateral chronic papilledema in a 24-year-old woman with pseudotumor cerebri. Note the glistening white bodies, which have been referred to as "pseudodrusen."

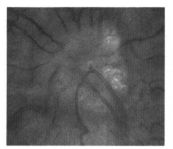

OD

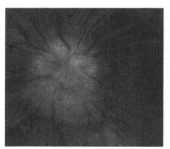

OS

10. Chronic papilledema in a 24-year-old woman with pseudotumor cerebri. Note disk pallor OD and the asymmetry of the disk edema. This asymmetry is due to damage to the right optic nerve.

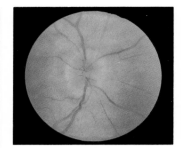

OD

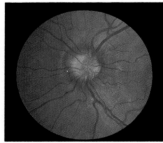

OS

11. Bilateral optic disk edema in a 40-year-old man with malignant hypertension.

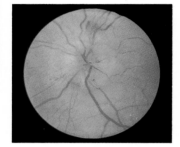

OD

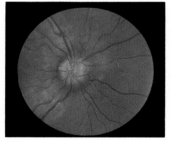

OS

12. Pseudopapilledema in a 12-year-old boy. Note that although the margins of the disk are irregular, the nerve fiber layer appears normal.

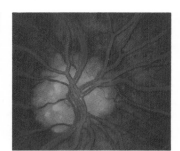

OD

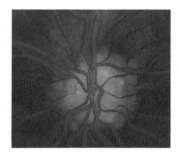

OS

13. Optic disk drusen OU in a 23-year-old man.

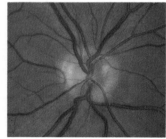

OD

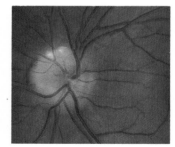

OS

14. Optic disk drusen OU with ischemic optic neuropathy OS in a 25-year-old woman. Note the swelling of the superior disk OS.

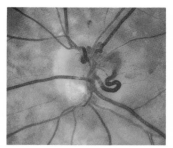

15. Optic disk edema OS with optociliary shunt vessels in a 42-year-old woman with a sphenoid meningioma.

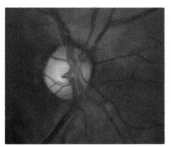

OD

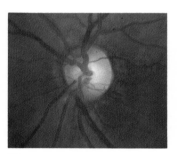

OS

16. Temporal optic disk pallor OU in a 7-year-old boy with dominant optic atrophy.

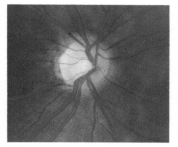

OD

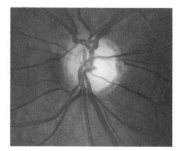

OS

17. Temporal optic disk pallor OU in an 11-year-old girl with recessive optic atrophy associated with diabetes mellitus.

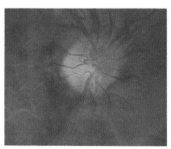

OD

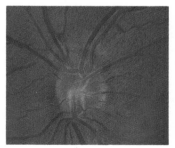

OS

18. Leber's optic atrophy in a 26-year-old man. Note the hyperemia of the superior portion of the right disk and the hyperemia of the disk in the asymptomatic left eye. Note the fullness of the peripapillary nerve fiber layer in both eyes. Telangiectatic vessels were present at the edge of the left disk.

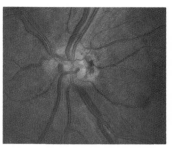

19. Optic nerve hypoplasia in the left eye of a 9-month-old boy. The right disk appeared similar.

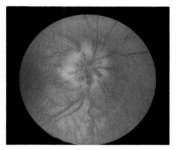

20. Optic disk coloboma OS in a 50-year-old man.

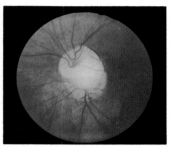

21. Papillophlebitis OD in a 23-year-old woman.

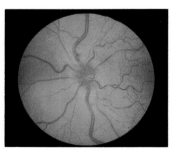

22. Partial central retinal vein occlusion OS in an asymptomatic 55-year-old woman. Note the marked hyperemia of the left disk and dilation of the retinal veins.

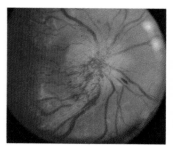

OD

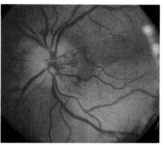

OS

23. Bilateral optic disk edema in a 17-year-old girl with juvenile diabetes mellitus. Note the prominent telangiectatic vessels overlying the disk surface.

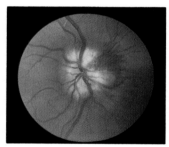

24. Swelling of the right optic disk in a 30-year-old man with sarcoidosis. Note the whitish nature of the disk swelling.

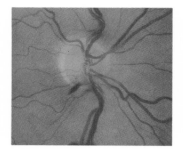

OD

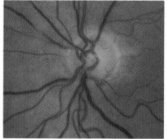

OS

25. Optic disk infarct—6:45 syndrome in both eyes of a 70-year-old woman. Note the cupping of the left optic disk to the rim inferiorly and the hemorrhage at the edge of the right disk inferiorly.

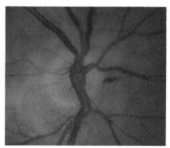

OD

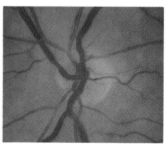

OS

26. Bilateral optic disk edema in a 67-year-old woman following severe blood loss.

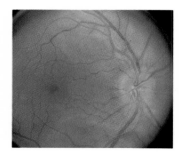

OD

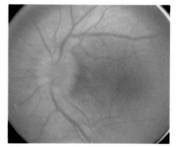

OS

27. Bilateral optic disk edema and vitritis in a 45-year-old man with syphilis.

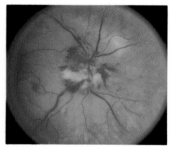

28. Hemorrhagic optic disk swelling OD in a 66-year-old man as the result of radiation given one year earlier for a sinus carcinoma.

5

Giant Cell Arteritis

A 72-year-old woman presented for consultation 1 day after sudden loss of vision in the left eye. She had been feeling ill for about 3 months with weakness, reduced appetite, a 15-lb weight loss, intermittent headaches, and occasional pain in her jaw. She had seen her family physician on several occasions, but no diagnosis was established. Her medical history was remarkable for a colectomy 20 years earlier for colon cancer.

Neuro-Ophthalmic Examination

	OD	OS
Visual acuity	20/20	20/25
Color plates correct	10 of 10	8 of 10
Pupils		Relative afferent pupillary defect
Motility, lids, orbits	Normal	Normal
Fundi	Normal	Swollen optic disk, one retinal cotton-wool spot (see Plate 6)

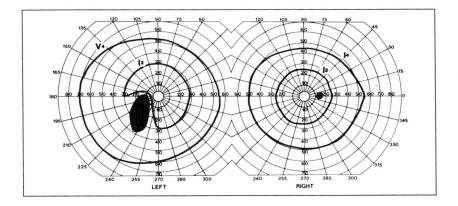

Summary

A 72-year-old woman with 3 months of multiple systemic symptoms developed sudden visual loss in the left eye and on examination was found to have slightly reduced visual acuity, a visual field defect, a pale swollen optic disk, and one retinal cotton-wool spot in the left eye.

Differential Diagnosis

Visual loss associated with optic disk edema in this age group is probably secondary to anterior ischemic optic neuropathy (AION). As discussed in Chapter 4, AION may be due to giant cell arteritis or may be classified as idiopathic. In this patient, the presence of systemic symptoms and the cotton-wool spot observed in the retina both strongly suggest arteritis. The relatively mild nature of the visual deficit is more typical of nonarteritic AION, however. A compressive lesion would be extremely unlikely in this patient and need not be considered further at this point. Optic neuritis at this age is only a remote possibility. Infiltration from a malignant process is the most likely alternate cause; if further workup did not confirm arteritis as the cause, computed tomography, lumbar puncture, and a systemic evaluation for malignancy might be indicated.

Clinical Diagnosis: Giant Cell Arteritis Producing Anterior Ischemic Optic Neuropathy

Giant cell arteritis is a systemic disorder occurring primarily in the over-60 age group in whom ocular changes are common. A multitude of systemic symptoms including headache, muscle weakness, myalgias, joint pain in shoulder and hip girdles, jaw claudication, fever, malaise, weight loss, and depression, are possible, often preceding ocular involvement by months. Unfortunately the diagnosis is frequently delayed, as it was in this case, because of the vague nature of many of these complaints.

AION is the most common ocular manifestation of giant cell arteritis. Autopsy studies have demonstrated that occlusion of the posterior ciliary arteries by the arteritic process is the cause. In the usual patient, visual loss occurs suddenly in one or both eyes and is severe. Progression of visual loss is much more common in arteritic than in nonarteritic AION. Transient visual phenomena, either a blackout of vision or flashing lights, lasting seconds to minutes may precede the development of arteritic AION. If a history of such occurrences is elicited from the patient with AION, giant cell arteritis should be strongly considered since preceding amaurosis fugax is extremely rare in nonarteritic AION. See Table 4-1 for a summary of the features that differentiate arteritic from nonarteritic AION.

Acutely the optic disk is swollen in arteritic as it is in nonarteritic AION. It is often not possible to separate these two conditions based on disk appearance, but a chalky white disk appearance is particularly characteristic of arteritis. Concomitant retinal ischemia, as present in this case, is also highly suggestive of arteritis.

Vision that is lost is virtually never recovered. The disk edema usually resolves within several weeks, and optic atrophy ensues. Marked cupping may occur, in contrast to nonarteritic AION in which cupping usually does not develop. Other ocular manifestations of giant cell arteritis occur less commonly: amaurosis fugax; retinal infarction—cotton-wool spots, branch retinal artery occlusion, central retinal artery occlusion;

anterior segment or extraocular muscle ischemia; ophthalmic artery occlusion with signs of both anterior and posterior segment ischemia; ocular motor nerve palsies; and retrobulbar ischemic optic neuropathy. Retrobulbar ischemic optic neuropathy is an extremely rare condition, but when it does occur, vasculitis—collagen vascular disease in younger patients, giant cell arteritis in older ones—is the most likely cause.

Additional Testing

An erythrocyte sedimentation rate (ESR) should be obtained in all cases of suspected giant cell arteritis. The Westergren method is more reliable than the Wintrobe or Zeta. Many patients with giant cell arteritis have a Westergren ESR greater than 100 mm per hour, but values greater than 40 mm per hour should be considered suspicious. In up to 5 percent of cases of giant cell arteritis, however, the ESR is normal (see Chapter 4).

A superficial temporal artery biopsy is the only way to establish a definitive diagnosis of giant cell arteritis and should be performed whenever the diagnosis is suspected, except perhaps when clinical evidence for arteritis is overwhelming. (Even then we tend to perform a biopsy.) As large a specimen as possible should be obtained since areas of normal artery (skip areas) may be interspersed with areas of diseased artery. Routine histopathologic staining and light microscopy are usually sufficient for diagnosis although special stains and electron microscopy may be useful in some cases. It is generally not necessary to perform a biopsy on both sides. A reasonable approach is to do a biopsy on one side and if the diagnosis remains equivocal then consider biopsy of the other side.

In a small percentage of cases of arteritis, the superficial temporal artery biopsy specimen will appear normal. Thus with strong clinical evidence, a diagnosis of arteritis should still be entertained even when the biopsy specimen is normal.

Treatment

Systemic corticosteroids are of unequivocal value in the management of giant cell arteritis to quiet the inflammatory response and prevent additional visual loss. Therapy should be instituted as soon as the diagnosis is considered and not deferred until after a temporal artery biopsy is performed. Histologic changes will not be altered by the corticosteroids if the biopsy is performed within a week or perhaps even longer. If after the biopsy results are obtained, the diagnosis of giant cell arteritis seems remote, then the corticosteroids can be discontinued. There is no uniformity of opinion regarding the proper dosage of corticosteroids. The dosage must be individualized, but starting doses are generally in the range of 60 to 150 mg of prednisone in cases with ocular involvement. Several days of high-dose intravenous corticosteroid therapy (1 gm methylprednisolone per day) should be considered in patients with visual loss of less than 48 hours' duration, especially when involvement has been bilateral. Most patients with arteritis will have dramatic improvement in their systemic symptoms within a few days of commencing therapy. Cortico-steroids are generally tapered over a 1- to 2-year period, with monitoring of clinical symptoms and signs as well as the ESR. Daily rather than alternate-day therapy is generally prescribed.

Other chemotherapeutic agents have been tried in the treatment of giant cell arteritis but have not proved to be of value.

Management and Course of the Case

A Westergren ESR was 102 mm per hour. Because the patient's visual loss had been of less than 48 hours' duration, she was hospitalized and given intravenous methylprednisolone (250 mg every 6 hours). Unfortunately she lost further vision over the next 24-hour period to the level of hand motion in the left eye. The right eye remained normal. Intravenous treatment was continued for 3 days, and she was discharged on a regimen of 100 mg of oral prednisone per day. Even though a diagnosis of giant cell arteritis seemed unequivocal, a temporal artery biopsy was performed and confirmed the diagnosis. Her systemic symptoms resolved after 2 days of steroid treatment and there was no further visual loss. The prednisone was reduced to 80 mg daily after 2 weeks, at which time the ESR was 37 mm per hour. After 1 month optic disk edema had resolved and optic atrophy ensued with moderate cupping of the disk. The prednisone was gradually tapered over a period of 1½ years.

Giant Cell Arteritis with Bilateral AION

A 69-year-old man noted progressive visual loss in the left eye over a period of 2 weeks. He had not noted any problems with the right eye. He had a dull headache but otherwise felt well.

Visual acuity was 20/20 in the right eye and 20/400 in the left eye. A left relative afferent pupillary defect was present. The left optic disk had diffuse pallid swelling. The disk in the asymptomatic right eye was swollen superiorly (see Plate 7). His visual field is shown below.

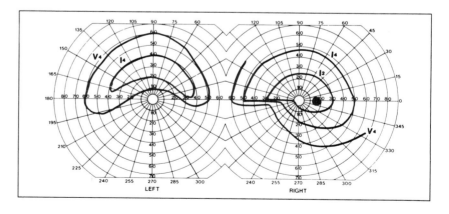

Although the patient was asymptomatic in the right eye, he had optic disk edema and a visual field defect in that eye. A picture of bilateral simultaneous AION is usually due to giant cell arteritis. The ESR was 85 mm per hour. A left superficial temporal artery biopsy confirmed giant cell arteritis as the diagnosis. When arteritic AION occurs, it is bilateral in approximately 50 percent of cases.

Bibliography

Albert, D. M., Searl, S. S., and Craft, J. L. Histologic and ultrastructural characteristics of temporal arteritis: The value of the temporal artery biopsy. *Ophthalmology* 89:1111, 1982.

Bengtsson, B. A., and Malmvall, B. E. The epidemiology of giant cell arteritis including temporal arteritis and polymyalgia rheumatica. *Arthritis Rheum.* 24:899, 1981.

Brennan, J., and McCrary, J. A. Diagnosis of superficial temporal arteritis. *Ann. Ophthalmol.* 7:1125, 1975.

Cullen, J. F., and Coleiro, J. A. Ophthalmic complications of giant cell arteritis. *Surv. Ophthalmol.* 20:247, 1976.

Goodwin, J. A. Temporal Arteritis. In P. J. Vinken and G. W. Bruyn (eds.), *The Handbook of Clinical Neurology,* Vol. 39. Amsterdam: Elsevier–North Holland, 1980.

Kansu, T., et al. Giant cell arteritis with normal sedimentation rate. *Arch. Neurol.* 34:624, 1977.

Keltner, J. L. Giant cell arteritis: Signs and symptoms. *Ophthalmology* 89:1101, 1982.

Wilkinson, I. M. S., and Russell, R. W. R. Arteries of the head and neck in giant cell arteritis: A pathological study to show the pattern of arterial involvement. *Arch. Neurol.* 27:378, 1972.

6

Pseudotumor Cerebri

A 21-year-old woman described a 2-month history of worsening head-aches; blackouts of vision for seconds in one or both eyes, usually on standing; and, more recently, horizontal diplopia, worse in the distance than near.

She was 5 ft 2 in. tall and weighed 187 lb. Her medical history was unremarkable.

Neuro-Ophthalmic Examination

	OD	OS
Visual acuity	20/20	20/20
Color plates correct	10 of 10	10 of 10
Pupils	Normal	Normal
Motility	Normal	50% abduction
Lids, orbits	Normal	Normal
Fundi (see Plate 8)	Swollen optic disk	Swollen optic disk

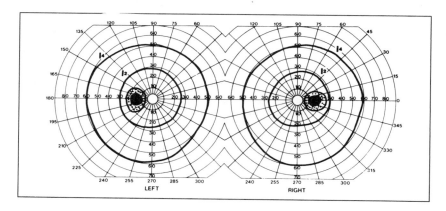

A neurologic examination was normal.

Summary

A 21-year-old overweight woman with headaches, diplopia, and tran-sient visual obscurations was found to have bilateral optic disk edema, increased blind spots on visual field testing, normal visual acuity, and a left abduction deficit.

58

Differential Diagnosis

Bilateral optic disk edema in association with normal optic nerve function is almost always due to increased intracranial pressure. In this setting it is called papilledema. The abduction deficit is almost certainly due to a sixth nerve palsy, which is also common with increased intracranial pressure. In a young overweight woman who has no focal neurologic signs, pseudotumor cerebri is the most likely diagnosis. Other causes of increased intracranial pressure to consider include brain tumor, meningitis, and a venous sinus thrombosis. Rarely aqueductal stenosis or other causes of hydrocephalus may be present. A marked elevation of blood pressure could produce the clinical picture of bilateral optic disk edema with normal optic nerve function as well as the headache but would not be expected to produce the diplopia or transient visual obscurations. If a diagnosis of increased intracranial pressure were not confirmed with additional testing, other disorders to consider in which optic disk edema may be accompanied by normal optic nerve function include diabetic papillopathy, sarcoidosis, papillophlebitis, partial central retinal vein occlusion, superior vena cava obstruction, pickwickian syndrome, and syphilis (see Chapter 16).

Of course it is necessary to ascertain that the patient has true rather than pseudopapilledema. This distinction can almost always be made on clinical grounds, as described in Chapter 7.

Clinical Diagnosis: Increased Intracranial Pressure, Probably Caused by Pseudotumor Cerebri

Pseudotumor cerebri is a clinical syndrome of unknown cause characterized by an increase in intracranial pressure, with no evidence of a mass lesion on neuroradiologic studies and a normal cerebrospinal fluid (CSF) composition. It is postulated that there is a reduction in cerebrospinal fluid outflow, but the mechanism of this reduction is unknown. The development of pseudotumor cerebri has been associated with vitamin A intoxication, tetracycline therapy, steroid withdrawal, intracranial venous sinus thrombosis, internal jugular occlusion, systemic lupus erythematosus, and renal failure, but in most cases a precipitating factor is not apparent. Associations with endocrine dysfunction appear to be chance.

The disorder is most common in obese females in the childbearing years. Presenting symptoms, which include headache, diplopia, transient visual obscurations, and blurred vision, vary from patient to patient. Some patients do not experience headache despite greatly increased intracranial pressure. Transient visual obscurations represent a temporary reduction in blood flow to the eye but do not correlate with impending optic nerve damage. Other less common complaints include the hearing of a noise in the head, facial pain, and neck pain.

Except in rare cases the papilledema is bilateral, although it may be asymmetric. The subarachnoid space extends the entire length of the optic nerve up to the lamina cribrosa, and with increased intracranial pressure disk edema results from the blockage of axoplasmic flow within the nerve. This leads to an increase in intraaxonal volume but not extracellular fluid volume. The appearance of papilledema varies depending on the duration and severity of the elevation of intracranial pressure. Acutely the disk is elevated and hyperemic. The retinal veins may be dilated, and hemorrhages and exudates may be present. In chronic cases the venous distention and hemorrhages abate, and although the disk remains elevated the blurring in the nerve fiber layer may become less. The disk may take on a glistening appearance, and white deposits that have been called *pseudodrusen* may be noted. If nerve fiber damage occurs, disk pallor develops and disk elevation lessens. Since the disk edema represents obstipation of axoplasmic flow, the more nerve fibers that are damaged, the less disk elevation is present. With severe nerve damage there is no edema and a very pale flat disk is seen. Other funduscopic changes occasionally seen with papilledema include chorioretinal folds, optociliary shunt vessels, and subretinal neovascularization and hemorrhage.

Diplopia when present is almost always the result of unilateral or bilateral sixth nerve palsies. Involvement of the sixth nerve is a nonlocalizing sign of increased intracranial pressure and is thought to occur because of stretching of the nerve as it takes a sharp turn across the edge of the petrous ridge of the temporal bone. In rare cases third and fourth nerve palsies and skew deviation have been reported.

Optic nerve damage is generally considered to be the only serious adverse effect of pseudotumor cerebri. Serious visual loss may occur in as many as 25 percent of patients. Early, the only visual field defect is generally enlargement of the blind spot. The size of the blind spot depends on the extent of involvement of the peripapillary retina with edema and is not a sign of optic nerve damage. Visual field defects that develop are usually in a nerve fiber bundle distribution (see Chapter 1). Inferior nasal defects are most common. The central 5 degrees of the field are usually not involved early, and thus visual acuity generally remains normal until optic nerve damage is extensive. Occasionally visual acuity may be decreased because the optic disk edema has extended from the disk to involve the macula. It is imperative that this situation be differentiated from decreased acuity caused by optic nerve damage by observing the extent of the edema ophthalmoscopically and by noting on the visual field the enlargement of the blind spot up to central fixation.

Additional Testing

Any patient considered to have increased intracranial pressure should have an immediate workup. A computed tomography (CT) or magnetic resonance imaging scan is necessary to rule out a mass lesion. Ventricle size is usually normal or small. A lumbar puncture is the next step to confirm increased intracranial pressure and to rule out meningitis. Intracranial pressure of less than 200 mm of water should be considered normal, 200 to 250 mm of water borderline, and greater than 250 mm of water abnormal. If a normal intracranial pressure is found on lumbar puncture, it is possible that the patient experiences fluctuations in the pressure and that at other times it is increased. If increased intracranial pressure is confirmed and results of the other studies are normal, a diagnosis of pseudotumor cerebri can be made.

Management

Since visual loss is the only serious adverse effect of pseudotumor cerebri, patients should be followed with frequent, careful perimetry. All obese patients should be encouraged to begin a weight-reduction diet since weight loss seems to help in many cases. Loss of visual field is the only absolute indication for treatment.

In the patient with normal optic nerve function in whom visual symptoms and headaches are minimal, it is reasonable just to follow the patient without therapy. If the visual field is abnormal or headaches or transient visual obscurations are frequent, therapy to lower intracranial pressure should be instituted. Several options are available—serial lumbar punctures for several days, corticosteroids, and diuretics. There has not been a prospective clinical trial comparing the various therapeutic modalities. Our initial therapy is generally with diuretics, which work by reducing CSF production. Treatment is begun with acetazolamide (Diamox) in dosages of 1 to 2 gm per day. If this is not tolerated because of side effects (numbness in hands and feet and gastrointestinal symptoms most commonly), furosemide (Lasix) (80–120 mg/day) is substituted. We generally do not advocate serial lumbar punctures as they are often difficult to perform because of the patient's obesity and are poorly tolerated by the patient. However, in some cases this therapy is successful, presumably by creating a rent in the dura and thus a shunt. We also do not generally commence with corticosteroids as an initial therapy. Although this treatment generally will lower intracranial pressure and improve symptoms, in most patients intracranial pressure becomes elevated again on withdrawal of treatment, necessitating chronic therapy and exposing the patient to serious adverse side effects. If diuretic therapy is successful, a gradual taper of the medication can be prescribed over a period of several months. In the patient without evidence of optic nerve damage, perimetry should be checked monthly for a few months and then, if it remains normal, every 3 months until there is no apparent reelevation of intracranial pressure when therapy is discontinued.

An alternative to intracranial-pressure-reducing therapy in the patient with a normal visual field and headaches is to treat with a beta blocker or amitriptyline. This therapy is often successful in alleviating the headaches.

In the patient in whom visual field loss is present on the initial examination or develops during follow-up, aggressive treatment and frequent perimetry are necessary. Many optic nerve fibers must be damaged before visual field loss is apparent on the Goldmann perimeter (with standard testing), and thus early visual field loss generally indicates serious optic nerve damage. Static perimetry often shows defects that manual kinetic perimetry does not. Once the optic nerve has sustained major damage, visual loss can be quite rapid. If there is serious visual loss in one or both eyes on the initial examination or if visual field loss progresses despite medical therapy, surgery should be considered. The most widely used procedures are the lumbar-peritoneal shunt and optic nerve sheath decompression. The latter procedure has gained more widespread use in the last few years and is now our procedure of choice when surgery is indicated. In this procedure a window is cut in the optic nerve sheath through a lateral or medial orbitotomy. Results have been excellent and the failure rate low. After this procedure intracranial pressure remains elevated but the papilledema abates, presumably because the surgery acts to reduce the effect of the pressure on the nerve distal to the window that has been created. Our experience with lumbar-peritoneal shunting has not been as good. The complication and failure rates have been much higher, but we do consider this procedure in a patient with intractable headaches or in whom optic nerve sheath decompression fails.

Pseudotumor cerebri is not as self-limited a disease as some of the early literature has suggested. Although symptoms may improve and papilledema may resolve, intracranial pressure may still be elevated years later.

Management and Course of the Case

The patient was placed on a regimen of Diamox 500 mg four times a day and a weight-reduction diet. After 2 weeks her headaches and diplopia were improved. Papilledema remained in both eyes, but her visual field was still normal (except for enlargement of the blind spots). She was then followed monthly, and after 2 months disk edema had resolved and she was symptom free. She had lost 10 pounds. The Diamox was tapered over a 4-month period, and she has remained asymptomatic in 1 year of follow-up. She continued to lose weight and after 1 year weighed 25 pounds less than she had at the onset.

Pseudotumor Cerebri Treated with Optic Nerve Sheath Decompressions

A 24-year-old woman was diagnosed as having pseudotumor cerebri 6 months before our examination and was treated with corticosteroids and Diamox. Her visual field at that time and 3 months later was normal. She initially improved with therapy, but headaches and papilledema worsened whenever the corticosteroids were tapered. She was referred for evaluation.

Visual acuity was 20/20 in each eye, but visual field defects (see below) and chronic disk edema (see Plate 9) were present in each eye.

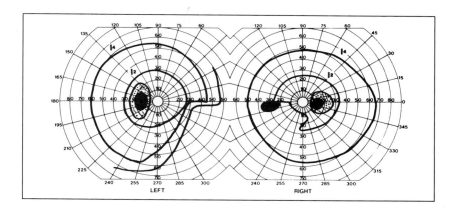

A lumbar puncture showed intracranial pressure to be 390 mm of water. Although visual field loss was mild, her optic disk appearance and history suggested chronic increased intracranial pressure. As mentioned above, visual field defects generally do not develop until serious optic nerve damage has occurred. Since the visual field loss had occurred despite medical therapy, optic nerve sheath decompressions were performed first on one side and then several days later on the other. Disk edema resolved over a 2-month period. The visual field in the right eye improved to normal, but there was no change in the field in the left eye. Amitriptyline 50 mg at bedtime was prescribed and relieved her headaches.

Pseudotumor Cerebri with Progressive Visual Loss

A 24-year-old woman with pseudotumor cerebri diagnosed 6 months earlier was referred for evaluation. She had been treated with dexamethasone without benefit during that time but not a diuretic. Visual acuity was 20/30 in each eye. Visual field defects and chronic disk edema were present bilaterally. The right disk was pale superiorly (see Plate 10).

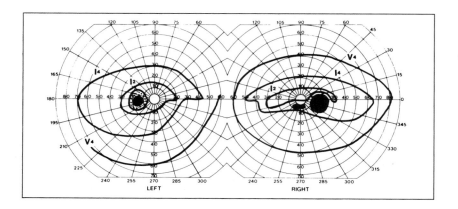

On lumbar puncture intracranial pressure was 550 mm of water. Diamox 500 mg four times a day was prescribed. On a return visit 10 days later her headaches were improved but vision was worse. Her visual field now showed extensive defects in each eye.

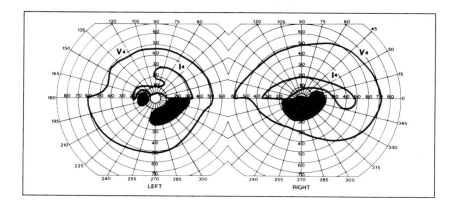

An emergency lumbar-peritoneal shunt was performed. It and two revisions failed, and vision further worsened. Two months later an optic nerve sheath decompression was performed in each eye. Her condition has remained stable for 2 years since then.

In retrospect the visual field defects present on her initial examination and the disk pallor in the right eye were signs of serious optic nerve damage. It would have been advisable to forgo further medical therapy at that point and perform optic nerve sheath decompressions.

Malignant Hypertension

Disk edema from malignant hypertension can appear identical to that from increased intracranial pressure. Plate 11 shows bilateral optic disk edema in a 40-year-old man with renal failure and a blood pressure of 210/120. Since he was not encephalopathic a CT scan and lumbar puncture were performed, with normal results.

Bibliography

Baker, R. S., et al. Visual loss in pseudotumor cerebri of childhood: A follow-up study. *Arch. Ophthalmol.* 103:1681, 1985.

Corbett, J. J. Problems in the diagnosis and treatment of pseudotumor cerebri. *Can. J. Neurol. Sci.* 10:221, 1983.

Corbett, J. J., and Mehta, M. P. Cerebrospinal fluid pressure in normal obese subjects and patients with pseudotumor cerebri. *Neurology* 33:1386, 1983.

Corbett, J. J., et al. Visual loss in pseudotumor cerebri: Follow-up of 57 patients from five to 41 years and a profile of 14 patients with permanent severe visual loss. *Arch. Neurol.* 39:461, 1982.

Couch, R., Camfield, P. R., and Tibbles, J. A. R. The changing picture of pseudotumor cerebri in children. *Can. J. Neurol. Sci.* 12:48, 1985.

Hayreh, S. S. Optic disc edema in raised intracranial pressure. *Arch. Ophthalmol.* 95:1553, 1977.

Keltner, J. L., et al. Optic nerve decompression: A clinical pathologic study. *Arch. Ophthalmol.* 95:97, 1977.

Orcutt, J. C., Page, N. G. R., and Sanders, M. D. Factors affecting visual loss in benign intracranial hypertension. *Ophthalmology* 91:1303, 1984.

Rush, J. A. Pseudotumor cerebri: Clinical profile and visual outcome in 63 patients. *Mayo Clin. Proc.* 55:541, 1980.

Sedwick, L. A., and Burde, R. M. Unilateral and asymmetric optic disk swelling with intracranial abnormalities. *Am. J. Ophthalmol.* 96:484, 1983.

Smith, C. H., and Orcutt, J. C. Surgical management of pseudotumor cerebri. *Int. Ophthalmol. Clin.* 26(4):265, 1986.

Wall, M., Hart, W. M., and Burde, R. M. Visual field defects in idiopathic intracranial hypertension (pseudotumor cerebri). *Am. J. Ophthalmol.* 96:654, 1983.

7

Pseudopapilledema

A 12-year-old boy was referred because of headaches and elevated optic disks. The headaches, which were often associated with nausea, were described as bifrontal and throbbing, occurring about once a week, lasting 1 to 4 hours, and generally relieved by sleep. He had no visual complaints. His medical history was otherwise unremarkable.

Neuro-Ophthalmic Examination

	OD	OS
Visual acuity	20/20	20/20
Color plates correct	10 of 10	10 of 10
Pupils	Normal	Normal
Motility, lids, orbits	Normal	Normal
Fundi (see Plate 12)	Elevated disk	Elevated disk

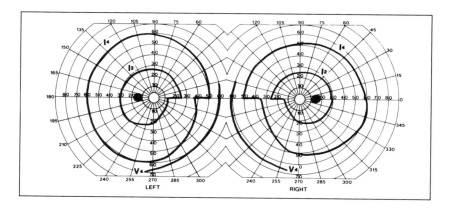

Results of a neurologic examination were normal.

Summary
A 12-year-old boy with headaches was found to have elevated optic disks and visual field defects but otherwise normal examination results.

Differential Diagnosis

In a case such as this, the clinician must determine whether the patient has true disk edema, which probably would be secondary to increased intracranial pressure, or whether the disk appearance is that of pseudopapilledema. Obviously the distinction is a crucial one since the diagnosis of true papilledema will indicate the urgent need for additional studies. In most cases the differentiation can be made with a high degree of certainty on clinical grounds.

If papilledema is well developed, the diagnosis is usually obvious. It is early papilledema that is difficult to distinguish from pseudopapilledema. Some of the distinguishing ophthalmoscopic features are summarized below.

Feature	Early papilledema	Pseudopapilledema
Disk color	Hyperemic	Pink, yellowish pink
Disk margins	Indistinct early at superior and inferior poles, later entire margin	Irregularly blurred, may be lumpy
Disk elevation	Minimal	Minimal to marked, center of disk most elevated
Vessels	Normal distribution, slight fullness, spontaneous venous pulsations absent	Emanate from center, frequent anomalous pattern, spontaneous venous pulsations present or absent
Nerve fiber layer	Dull owing to edema, which may obscure blood vessels	No edema, may glisten with circumpapillary halo of feathery light reflections
Hemorrhages	Splinter	Subretinal, retinal, vitreous

The appearance of the nerve fiber layer on the disk and at its margin is generally the one most useful distinguishing feature. In true papilledema the edema in the nerve fiber layer will generally obscure to some degree the underlying blood vessels, whereas in pseudopapilledema the vessels can be seen clearly. Venous distention and hemorrhages are possible in both and thus are not differentiating features. The presence of spontaneous venous pulsations would suggest pseudopapilledema, but as mentioned in Chapter 6 intracranial pressure can fluctuate between elevated and normal levels and thus the observation of spontaneous venous pulsations does not rule out an intracranial process.

In this case it can be seen in the photographs that although the disk margins were blurred, there was no obscuration of the underlying blood vessels and the nerve fiber layer was clear. Also the elevation of the disks was most prominent nasally in both eyes, particularly in the left. These features all suggest a diagnosis of pseudopapilledema. The headaches were probably migraine and were presumed to be unrelated to the disk anomaly.

Clinical Diagnosis: Pseudopapilledema

Pseudopapilledema is most commonly produced by optic disk drusen, although the drusen may be "buried" within the disk and not visible on the surface. High hyperopia with a small scleral canal and heaping up of the nerve fibers is another possible cause. Occasionally remnants of the embryologic hyaloid or myelination of the nerve fibers overlying the disk may be confused with disk edema.

Optic disk drusen are dominantly inherited with variable penetrance. The incidence is 20 in 1000, and they are present in whites much more commonly than in blacks. The pathogenesis of drusen has been postulated to be related to axonal degeneration from altered axoplasmic flow. The presence of drusen is usually an incidental finding, and not infrequently the observation of disk elevation is made in a patient being examined for a cause of headaches (as in this case). When on the surface of the disk, the drusen may be observed to be whitish and glistening. When buried they are not obvious, but the clinical features described above help to differentiate them from true papilledema. In children drusen tend to be buried, whereas in adults they are more often on the surface. The progression from buried to surface drusen in a given individual has been documented.

Optic disk drusen generally do not produce any visual symptoms although rarely a patient may experience transient visual obscurations similar to those with increased intracranial pressure. However, visual field defects are common, occurring in about 70 percent of eyes with visible drusen and 35 percent with pseudopapilledema but no visible drusen. The visual field defects are generally in a nerve fiber bundle distribution (see Chapter 1), with inferior nasal defects being most common. An increase in the blind spot and generalized field constriction are also possible. Progression of visual field defects is well documented. It is rare for visual acuity to be decreased from drusen, and if decreased visual acuity is noted in a patient with drusen, an evaluation for an alternative cause should be performed.

Visual loss can occur with drusen for reasons other than an effect on the optic nerve fibers: hemorrhage, retinal degeneration, or ischemic optic neuropathy. Hemorrhages with drusen are usually subretinal in a peripapillary distribution. Retinal and vitreous hemorrhages are less common. Retinitis pigmentosa occurs in association with drusen in about 2 percent of cases. Ischemic optic neuropathy occurs with a higher than expected frequency, especially in young adults.

Additional Testing and Management

If a clinical diagnosis of pseudopapilledema can be made with certainty, additional testing is not necessary. Fluorescein angiography is generally not helpful as there may be staining of the disk in both early papilledema and drusen. Ultrasound may be useful to identify buried drusen. If a diagnosis of pseudopapilledema is probable but not definite and the patient has no neurologic symptoms or signs, it is reasonable to photograph the disks and reexamine the patient in 1 to 2 months. If true papilledema is present some changes in the interim would be expected, whereas with pseudopapilledema the appearance should be identical.

If the diagnosis is in doubt, it is prudent to perform computed tomography to rule out an intracranial mass and, if the scan is normal, a lumbar puncture to measure intracranial pressure.

Management and Course of the Case

The clinical diagnosis of pseudopapilledema was felt to be definite. No further testing was performed. Treatment for migraine was recommended.

Optic Disk Drusen and Pituitary Tumor

A 23-year-old man with a pituitary tumor was found to have optic disk elevation and visual field defects in both eyes. Visual acuity was 20/20 in each eye.

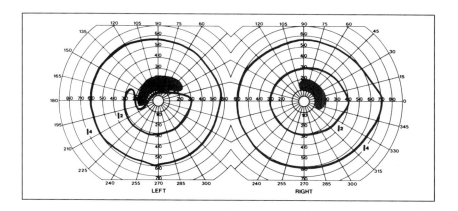

The patient has obvious drusen in both disks (see Plate 13) and the visual field defects are consistent with drusen as the cause. The pituitary tumor was presumed to be unrelated since the field defects do not suggest chiasmal involvement.

Optic Disk Drusen and Anterior Ischemic Optic Neuropathy

A 25-year-old woman experienced sudden visual loss in the left eye. Visual acuity was 20/20 in both eyes. Both optic disks had the appearance of drusen, but the left disk was also swollen superiorly and a visual field defect was present in the left eye (see Plate 14). The field in the right eye was normal.

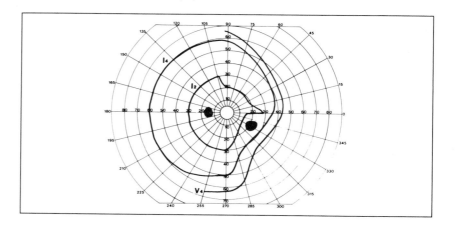

A diagnosis of anterior ischemic optic neuropathy with optic disk drusen was made. No treatment was instituted. The disk edema resolved over a 1-month period. The field defect remained unchanged. Note the subretinal hemorrhage at the left disk margin in the photograph. This is the most typical hemorrhage associated with drusen.

Optic Disk Drusen with Progressive Visual Loss

A 30-year-old woman noted visual loss in the right eye and 1 year later in the left eye. Over the next 20 years visual loss progressed in both eyes. Optic disk drusen were apparent in both eyes. The retina appeared normal.

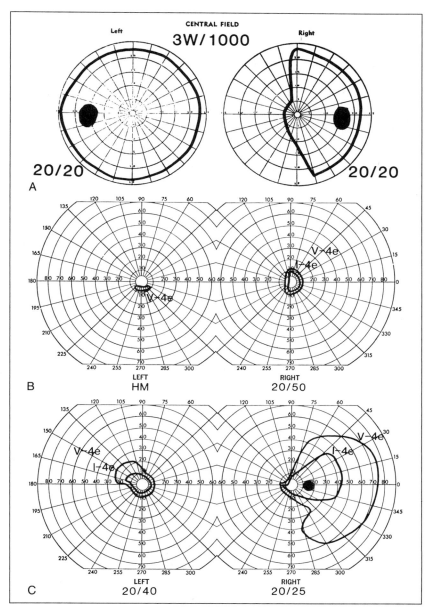

A. Visual field on tangent screen in 1961. B. Perimetry in 1978. C. Perimetry in 1983. (From R. W. Beck, et al. Decreased visual acuity from optic disc drusen. Arch. Ophthalmol. *August 1985, 103 : 1155. Copyright 1985, American Medical Association. With permission.)*

Results of extensive neuroradiologic evaluations and electroretinography were normal. The visual loss was presumed to be related to the drusen. Note that visual acuity remained normal until visual field loss was severe.

This degree of visual loss is rare but can occur from drusen. Diagnosis of drusen as a cause of severe visual loss should always be one of exclusion.

Bibliography

Beck, R. W., et al. Decreased visual acuity from optic disc drusen. *Arch. Ophthalmol.* 103:1155, 1985.

Erkkila, H. Optic disc drusen in children. *Acta Ophthalmol. [Suppl. 129] (Copenh.)* 55:7, 1977.

Lorentzen, S. E. Drusen of the optic disk. *Acta Ophthalmol. [Suppl. 90] (Copenh.)* 44:9, 1966.

Mustonen, E. Pseudopapilledema with and without verified optic disc drusen: A clinical analysis: II. Visual fields. *Acta Ophthalmol. [Suppl.] (Copenh.)* 61:1057, 1983.

Rosenberg, M. A., Savino, P. J., and Glaser, J. S. A clinical analysis of pseudopapilledema: I. Population, laterality, acuity, refractive error, ophthalmoscopic characteristics and coincident disease. *Arch. Ophthalmol.* 97:65, 1979.

Sadun, A. A., Currie, J. N., and Lessell, S. Transient visual obscurations with elevated optic discs. *Ann. Neurol.* 16:489, 1984.

Savino, P. J., Glaser, J. S., and Rosenberg, M. A. A clinical analysis of pseudopapilledema: II. Visual field defects. *Arch. Ophthalmol.* 97:71, 1979.

Tso, M. O. M. Pathology and pathogenesis of drusen of the optic nervehead. *Ophthalmology* 88:1066, 1981.

8

Compressive Optic Neuropathy

A 45-year-old woman reported gradual worsening of vision in the right eye over a 5-year period. She had no other symptoms and was otherwise in good health.

Neuro-Ophthalmic Examination

	OD	OS
Visual acuity	Hand motion	20/20
Color plates correct	None	10 of 10
Pupils	Relative afferent pupillary defect	
Motility, lids, orbits	Normal	Normal
Optic disks	Diffuse pallor	Normal

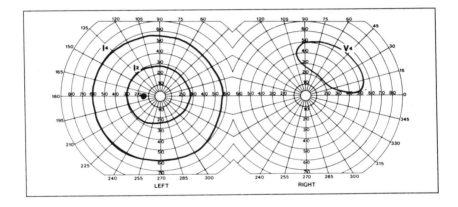

Summary

A 45-year-old woman with slowly progressive visual loss was found to have a marked decrease in vision, a relative afferent pupillary defect, and optic disk pallor in the right eye.

Differential Diagnosis

This patient has definite evidence of an optic neuropathy. With a history of gradual loss of vision, a compressive lesion is almost certain to be the diagnosis. The prolonged course suggests a benign process. All of the clinical findings could occur with optic neuritis or anterior ischemic optic neuropathy, but in both of these entities visual loss would be acute and not progressive over a long period. Since there was no proptosis and the visual field in the left eye was normal, it was not possible to localize the process to either the orbital or intracranial nerve (a superior temporal defect of the left eye would have indicated involvement of the posterior optic nerve; see Junctional Scotoma from Meningioma, below).

Meningioma is the most common mass to produce this clinical picture of a slowly progressive optic neuropathy. Optic nerve gliomas are extremely rare at this age and when present in adults usually produce rapid visual loss and death. Other possibilities include pituitary tumor, aneurysm, craniopharyngioma, and mucocele.

Clinical Diagnosis: Compressive Optic Neuropathy

As mentioned above a number of different lesions can produce compressive optic neuropathy. Pituitary tumors and craniopharyngiomas are discussed in Chapters 17 and 18. Aneurysms affecting the optic nerve most commonly arise from the internal carotid artery or ophthalmic artery. We review meningiomas in this chapter.

Meningiomas are the most common intracranial tumor. They arise from the meningothelial cells of the dural sheath and are almost always benign. Females are affected more commonly than males. The tumors are rare in childhood except in association with neurofibromatosis. Meningiomas affecting the optic nerve most commonly arise from the sphenoid wing, tuberculum sellae, planum sphenoidale, or the optic nerve sheath itself.

With sphenoid wing meningiomas the optic neuropathy is often accompanied by proptosis and impaired motility. If only the intracranial optic nerve is involved, the optic disk may appear normal or pale. With orbital involvement there is frequently swelling of the disk and optociliary shunt vessels may develop (see Optociliary Shunt Vessels from Meningioma, below).

Meningiomas arising from the tuberculum sellae or planum sphenoidale affect the posterior optic nerve and typically produce gradual loss of vision in one eye. The optic disk may appear pale but frequently appears normal, particularly if visual loss is not severe. Optic disk swelling is unusual. With these tumors, optic neuropathy is often the only sign.

Optic nerve sheath meningiomas typically produce gradual loss of vision over many years. Patients may note either decreased acuity or, occasionally, transient visual obscurations. Proptosis is present in the majority of patients but is not apparent in at least one-third of cases. Visual acuity may be normal or severely reduced at the time of presentation. Visual field defects vary considerably from patient to patient. In some there is a central scotoma early; in others there is considerable peripheral field loss before central fixation is affected. In comparison, decreased visual acuity and central scotomas are present in most patients with intracranial meningiomas affecting the optic nerve. As with sphenoid meningiomas, optic nerve sheath meningiomas frequently produce optic disk edema, and optociliary shunt vessels may develop. When the disk is swollen, yellow refractile bodies may be noted on the surface. In many cases of optic nerve sheath meningioma, visual loss is extremely slow and there may be little change over several years of follow-up. Bilateral optic nerve sheath meningiomas occasionally occur, particularly in association with neurofibromatosis.

Additional Testing and Management
Computed tomography (CT) or magnetic resonance imaging is likely to identify a compressive lesion in cases like this of a slowly progressive optic neuropathy.

INTRACRANIAL LESIONS
Intracranial meningiomas typically appear as contrast-enhancing masses. Calcification or hyperostosis may be noted. Craniopharyngiomas may be cystic or solid, and the degree of enhancement varies. The contrast-enhancing appearance of aneurysms may be quite similar to that of meningiomas, and in some cases a computed tomographic differentiation is not possible.

When the optic nerve is compromised from an intracranial meningioma or other neoplasm, surgical resection is usually indicated. An arteriogram is generally performed before surgery to assess the blood supply of the mass and differentiate it from aneurysm. Complete removal of a meningioma may not be possible, but usually the tumor can be debulked to relieve the compression of the optic nerve. Visual recovery varies considerably, but if optic atrophy is not present, recovery is often excellent.

INTRAORBITAL LESIONS
With an optic nerve sheath meningioma there is generally either a tubular thickening or fusiform enlargement of the optic nerve on computed tomography. Calcification in a ringlike pattern around the nerve is virtually pathognomonic but is not present in many cases. In most cases a diagnosis of optic nerve sheath meningioma can be made with a high degree of confidence based on the CT scan and clinical picture. In these cases if the tumor is confined to the orbit and vision is good, a reasonable approach is just to follow the patient without biopsy, unless the course becomes atypical, such as rapid visual loss, or intracranial extension is suggested. Yearly computed tomography should be performed to evaluate for signs of intracranial extension in those cases in which initial excision is not performed. It is possible to perform a biopsy on the lesion without producing further visual loss, but except in rare cases excision of the tumor does not restore vision and complete removal usually necessitates sacrificing the optic nerve. If canalicular or intracranial exten-

sion is noted, excision of the tumor should be strongly considered to prevent chiasmal involvement. When vision is reduced to hand motion or worse, we usually recommend excision of the tumor even when it appears to be confined to the orbit. Radiation therapy has been advocated for optic nerve sheath meningiomas, but because they are often so slow-growing, the response is usually poor. We generally reserve this treatment for bilateral cases.

If computed tomography fails to identify a compressive lesion yet one is still clinically suspected, a magnetic resonance imaging scan or, if not available, a metrizamide CT scan should be considered.

Management and Course of the Case

Computed tomography demonstrated diffuse enlargement of the intra-orbital optic nerve most consistent with optic nerve sheath meningioma.

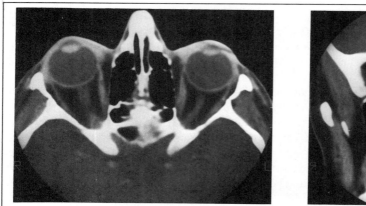

Axial

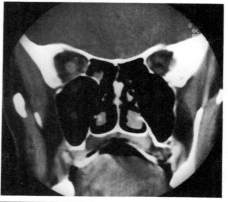

Coronal

Because virtually all vision had been lost in the right eye and because visual loss appeared to be more rapid than is typical for optic nerve sheath meningioma, we decided to resect the tumor. A diagnosis of meningioma was confirmed. An alternative approach would have been to follow the patient with periodic examinations and computed tomography and perform surgery only if the tumor began to extend intracranially.

Junctional Scotoma from Meningioma

A 50-year-old man who reported gradual visual loss in the right eye over a 1-year period was found on examination to have visual acuity of 20/80, dyschromatopsia, and a relative afferent pupillary defect in the right eye. Visual function in the left eye was normal. Both optic disks were pink. Results of perimetry are shown below.

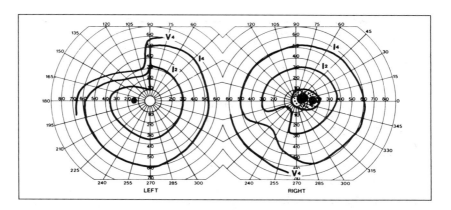

The visual field defect in the right eye is consistent with an optic neuropathy but does not help in localization. The superotemporal defect in the left eye indicates that the posterior optic nerve is the site of involvement and thus a compressive lesion is likely. Computed tomography demonstrated a mass, which at surgery was found to be a meningioma.

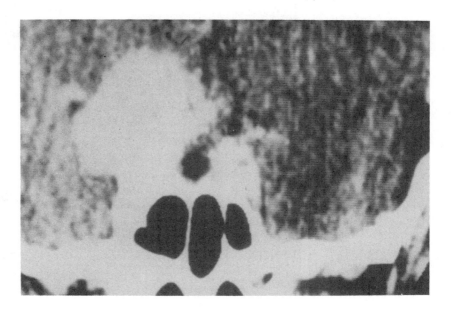

A 42-year-old woman who reported gradually worsening proptosis and vision in the left eye was found to have visual acuity of 20/400, a relative afferent pupillary defect, and 8 mm of proptosis in the left eye. The left optic disk was swollen with optociliary shunt vessels on the surface (see Plate 15). The right eye was normal. Perimetric results are shown below.

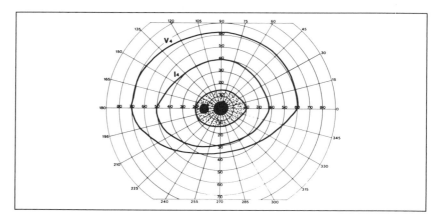

The presence of optic disk edema with optociliary shunt vessels and proptosis is highly suggestive of meningioma. Computed tomography demonstrated an enhancing mass with thickening of the sphenoid bone.

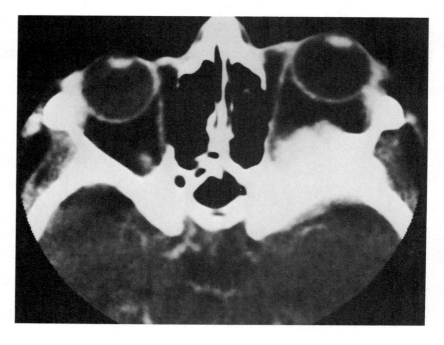

Although the patient refused surgery, the CT appearance and clinical findings are virtually pathognomonic of a meningioma. Optociliary shunts may also be seen in glaucoma, central retinal vein occlusion, malignant hypertension, and chronic papilledema and may be congenital.

Bibliography

Alper, M. G. Management of primary optic nerve meningiomas: Current status—therapy in controversy. *J. Clin. Neuro Ophthalmol.* 1:101, 1981.

Ehlers, N., and Malmros, R. The suprasellar meningioma: A review of the literature and presentation of a series of 31 cases. *Acta Ophthalmol. [Suppl.] (Copenh.)* 121:7, 1973.

Mark, L. E., et al. Microsurgical removal of a primary intraorbital meningioma. *Am. J. Ophthalmol.* 86:704, 1978.

Rosenberg, L. F., and Miller, N. R. Visual results after microsurgical removal of meningiomas involving the anterior visual system. *Arch. Ophthalmol.* 102:1019, 1984.

Sibony, P. A., et al. Intrapapillary refractile bodies in optic nerve sheath meningioma. *Arch. Ophthalmol.* 103:383, 1985.

Sibony, P. A., et al. Optic nerve sheath meningiomas: Clinical manifestations. *Ophthalmology* 91:1313, 1984.

Smith, J. L., et al. Radiation therapy for primary optic nerve meningiomas. *J. Clin. Neuro Ophthalmol.* 1:85, 1981.

9

Optic Glioma

A 6-year-old boy was examined because of decreased visual acuity. He was otherwise in good health. His history was unremarkable.

Neuro-Ophthalmic Examination

	OD	OS
Visual acuity	20/40	20/50
Color plates correct	Control only	Control only
Pupils	Normal	Normal
Motility, lids, orbits	Normal	Mass, left upper lid
Optic disks	Pale	Pale
Confrontation field	Normal	Normal

Results of a neurologic examination were normal. Physical examination showed multiple café au lait spots on the skin.

Summary

A 6-year-old boy with decreasing vision for 2 years was found to have reduced visual acuity and optic atrophy in both eyes as well as multiple café au lait spots and a soft mass in his left upper lid.

Differential Diagnosis

In view of the multiple café au lait spots, neurofibromatosis with a chiasmal or bilateral optic nerve glioma is almost certainly the diagnosis. Meningioma would also be possible but is less likely.

Clinical Diagnosis: Optic Nerve or Chiasmal Glioma with Neurofibromatosis

Optic nerve gliomas are generally histologically benign astrocytic proliferations. They are often associated with neurofibromatosis. These tumors occur mainly in children less than 10 and are rare in adults. Either the optic nerve or chiasm may be involved.

An intraorbital glioma produces gradual visual loss often in association with optic disk edema and progressive proptosis. Optociliary shunt vessels like those seen with meningiomas (see Chapter 8) may develop on the optic disk. Visual loss may be mild or severe. Bilateral optic nerve gliomas are highly suggestive of neurofibromatosis.

Chiasmal gliomas are also frequently associated with neurofibromatosis. Visual loss usually occurs in both eyes and again varies from mild to severe. At the time of presentation optic disk pallor is usually present even if vision is good. Nystagmus may be associated with chiasmal gliomas and may be confused with spasmus nutans. There also may be pituitary or hypothalamic dysfunction.

Approximately 10 percent of patients with neurofibromatosis have evidence of optic nerve or chiasmal glioma on computed tomography. These tumors are frequently asymptomatic, and vision is often normal.

Additional Testing

Generally a diagnosis of optic nerve or chiasmal glioma can be made with a high degree of accuracy with computed tomography (CT) or magnetic resonance imaging. Optic nerve gliomas can appear as either a diffuse or more typically a fusiform enlargement of the nerve. With a chiasmal glioma the optic chiasm appears several times larger than normal. In some patients with neurofibromatosis both optic nerves and the chiasm are enlarged. Optic tract involvement may also be seen.

In patients without known neurofibromatosis, a thorough family history and physical examination for stigmata of neurofibromatosis are necessary.

When a chiasmal glioma is found, pituitary and hypothalamic function studies should be performed.

Management

Treatment of optic nerve and chiasmal gliomas is controversial. Management varies to some degree dependent on whether neurofibromatosis is present.

In the patient with an intraorbital tumor presumed on clinical and radiologic grounds to be a glioma in whom neurofibromatosis is not present, consideration can be given to observation, biopsy, or excision. Biopsy may be warranted to confirm the diagnosis. Excision should be performed if visual loss is severe, particularly with disfiguring proptosis, but can be deferred in a patient with a classic CT appearance of optic nerve glioma in whom vision is good. In the patient with neurofibromatosis, biopsy is generally not necessary for diagnosis, and excision should be considered only if visual loss is severe and proptosis is disfiguring.

With a chiasmal tumor, biopsy is generally indicated in all patients without neurofibromatosis. In the patient with neurofibromatosis and a CT scan typical of chiasmal glioma, we generally do not recommend surgery for diagnosis and would consider it only if the tumor grew to such an extent that neurologic dysfunction occurred.

In cases of bilateral optic nerve or chiasmal glioma, visual function should be documented as well as possible, given the patient's age. We generally do not prescribe any treatment initially in patients in whom optic nerve or chiasmal involvement is the only impairment. Should there be progression of visual loss, radiation therapy or chemotherapy (vincristine sulfate and dactinomycin [actinomycin D]) can be considered. These tumors are usually extremely slow-growing and years may pass without major change in tumor size or visual function. This makes it very difficult to judge the efficacy of any therapy. Long-term survival in these patients is usually good.

Management and Course of the Case
A CT scan showed diffuse enlargement of both optic nerves and the chiasm.

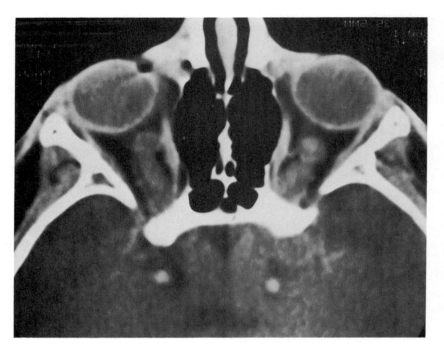

A diagnosis of neurofibromatosis with optic glioma was made. The mass in the lid was presumed to be a neurofibroma. An endocrinologic evaluation yielded normal results. The patient was observed without therapy for 1 year, but visual acuity decreased to 20/70 in the right eye and 20/100 in the left. Chemotherapy consisting of vincristine sulfate and dactinomycin was then started. Visual acuity remained stable for about the next 9 months, but then a decrease to 20/200 in each eye occurred. He then received radiation to the optic nerves and chiasm. Visual acuity has been stable in the subsequent 1 year. There has been no change in the CT appearance of the nerves from the initial scan.

Unilateral Optic Nerve Glioma

A 3-year-old girl's vision was found to be light perception in the right eye with a right relative afferent pupillary defect, mild proptosis, and a pale swollen optic disk. The left eye was normal. An optic nerve glioma was suspected and confirmed on computed tomography. There were no signs of neurofibromatosis. Because visual loss in the right eye was already severe, a decision was made to resect the tumor, which proved to be a glioma.

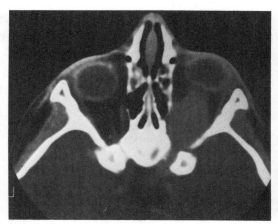

Axial

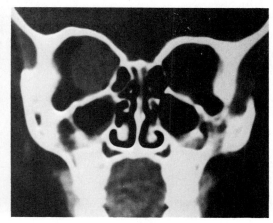

Coronal

Bibliography

Danoff, B. J., Kramer, S., and Thompson, N. The radiotherapeutic management of optic nerve gliomas in children. *Int. J. Radiat. Oncol. Biol. Phys.* 6:45, 1980.

Horwich, A., and Bloom, H. J. G. Optic gliomas: Radiation therapy and prognosis. *Int. J. Radiat. Oncol. Biol. Phys.* 11:1067, 1985.

Hoyt, W. F., and Baghdassarian, S. A. Optic gliomas of childhood: Natural history and rationale for conservative management. *Br. J. Ophthalmol.* 53:793, 1969.

Imes, R. K., and Hoyt, W. F. Childhood chiasmal gliomas: Update on the fare of patients in the 1969 study. *Br. J. Ophthalmol.* 70:179, 1986.

Lewis, R. A., et al. von Recklinghausen neurofibromatosis: II. Incidence of optic gliomata. *Ophthalmology* 91:929, 1984.

Packer, R. J., et al. Chiasmatic gliomas of childhood: A reappraisal of natural history and effectiveness of cranial irradiation. *Childs Brain* 10:393, 1983.

Rosenstock, J. G., et al. Chiasmatic optic glioma treated with chemotherapy: A preliminary report. *J. Neurosurg.* 63:862, 1985.

Rush, J. A., et al. Optic glioma: Long-term follow-up of 85 histopathologically verified cases. *Ophthalmology* 89:1213, 1982.

Spoor, T. C., et al. Malignant gliomas of the optic nerve pathways. *Am. J. Ophthalmol.* 89:284, 1980.

Stern, J., Jakobiec, F. A., and Housepian, E. M. The architecture of optic nerve gliomas with and without neurofibromatosis. *Arch. Ophthalmol.* 98:505, 1980.

Tenny, R. T., et al. The neurosurgical management of optic glioma: Results in 104 patients. *J. Neurosurg.* 57:452, 1982.

10

Hereditary Optic Atrophy

A 7-year-old boy was found on a school eye examination to have decreased visual acuity in each eye. He had no visual symptoms. His history was unremarkable.

Neuro-Ophthalmic Examination

	OD	OS
Visual acuity	20/50	20/40
Color plates correct	7 of 9	7 of 9
Pupils	Normal	Normal
Motility, lids, orbits	Normal	Normal
Fundi (see Plate 16)	Temporal optic disk pallor	Temporal optic disk pallor

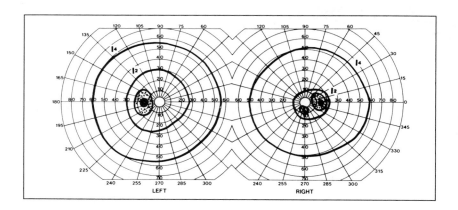

Neurologic examination was normal.

Summary
A 7-year-old boy with no visual symptoms was found to have visual acuity of 20/50 in the right eye and 20/40 in the left with mild dyschromatopsia and optic disk pallor in both eyes.

Differential Diagnosis

The most common causes of a bilateral optic neuropathy are hereditary afflictions, poor nutrition, vitamin B_{12} or folate deficiencies, tobacco-alcohol amblyopia, drugs, and toxins (e.g., heavy metals). A compressive lesion is unlikely since the visual loss does not suggest chiasmal involvement, but bilateral optic nerve tumors are possible, particularly in neurofibromatosis. Bilateral optic neuritis is also possible, but an insidious onset would be atypical. Asymptomatic optic nerve demyelination can occur in multiple sclerosis, but this would be an extremely rare presenting sign for the disease.

Additional History

Since by history and examination there were no indications of a toxic or nutritional cause, a diagnosis of hereditary (dominant) optic atrophy was considered. Examination of the patient's 15-year-old brother, 40-year-old father, and his father's 36-year-old brother disclosed bilateral temporal disk pallor in each, with visual acuities ranging from 20/25 to 20/40.

Clinical Diagnosis: Dominant Optic Atrophy

There are several forms of hereditary optic neuropathy, which may follow a mendelian (dominant or recessive) or nonmendelian (Leber's) inheritance pattern. The rarest is recessive optic atrophy, in which severe bilateral loss is generally the rule. One form of recessive optic atrophy has its onset in early infancy or childhood and may be associated with ataxia and other neurologic problems. Another form begins between ages 5 and 15 and may be associated with diabetes mellitus (see Recessive Optic Atrophy Associated with Juvenile Diabetes, below). Leber's optic atrophy is discussed in Chapter 11.

Dominant optic atrophy is by far the most common inherited optic nerve disorder. Visual loss usually has an insidious onset between ages 5 and 10. It is frequently asymptomatic and not uncommonly is first noted on a routine visual acuity test, as in this case. Visual loss varies from mild to moderate. Visual acuity may remain at 20/20 or be reduced as low as 20/200, but the majority of patients have visual acuity between 20/30 and 20/70. Only a rare patient will have visual acuity worse than 20/200. Although both eyes are always affected, the degree of involvement may be asymmetric. There is usually a loss of color perception, which may be generalized or predominantly along a tritan (yellow-blue) axis. Perimetry can usually demonstrate the presence of a central scotoma in each eye, but frequently the density of the scotoma is less than expected from the level of visual acuity. The reason for this is uncertain. With color targets it may be possible to demonstrate that the field to blue is smaller than the field to red (normally the blue field is larger than the red). The optic disks will generally appear pale temporally, although the degree of pallor varies. The pale temporal portion of the disk may also be excavated.

Patients with dominant optic atrophy generally do well from a visual standpoint. Visual loss may progress for a few years but usually remains stable after the teens. Patients usually do not seem as disabled by the decrease in acuity as do patients with loss of acuity to the same level from other causes. There are generally no associated neurologic abnormalities.

Additional Testing

A detailed family history should be taken and, when appropriate, other family members examined as in this case. Since visual loss may be mild, there may be affected family members who are not aware of a visual problem.

Color testing with the Farnsworth-Munsell 100-hue or 15-hue test is useful to try to define a yellow-blue axis of color loss, which, in a patient with an acquired optic neuropathy, is relatively specific for dominant optic atrophy.

Visual field testing using red and blue test objects can be performed to determine whether there is inversion of the isopters for the targets. Normally a field plotted with a blue target is larger than a field plotted with a red target, but in patients with dominant optic atrophy the blue field may be constricted.

In some cases the clinician may strongly suspect a diagnosis of dominant optic atrophy but may not be able to identify the abnormality in other family members (or they may be unavailable for examination). In these cases computed tomography should be performed to rule out the unusual possibility of a compressive lesion, and a vitamin deficiency, adverse drug effect, or toxin should be considered.

Management and Course of the Case

At age 9, Farnsworth-Munsell 100-hue testing showed the patient to have a general loss of color vision without a specific axis in either eye. In 6 additional years of follow-up, he remained asymptomatic, although vision decreased to 20/60 in both eyes. Since a diagnosis of dominant optic atrophy seemed firm based on the findings in other family members, no additional testing was prescribed.

He continued to function well in school with normal-size-print books and without any visual aid.

Recessive Optic Atrophy Associated with Juvenile Diabetes

An 11-year-old girl who had recently been diagnosed as having insulin-dependent diabetes mellitus gradually lost vision in both eyes. Visual acuity was 20/40, and disk pallor was noted in each eye (see Plate 17). One year later visual acuity was 20/60 in each eye, and a marked dyschromatopsia and a worsening of the disk pallor were noted. Despite these findings perimetric results were essentially normal.

Two of her six siblings also had diabetes mellitus and optic atrophy and one had diabetes mellitus alone. No other family members in earlier generations were known to be affected.

This case represents a recessively inherited form of optic atrophy associated with diabetes mellitus. In some cases deafness, diabetes insipidus, and, less commonly, other neurologic abnormalities are also associated.

Bibliography

Hoyt, C. S. Autosomal dominant optic atrophy: A spectrum of disability. *Ophthalmology* 87:245, 1980.

Johnston, P. B., et al. A clinicopathologic study of autosomal dominant optic atrophy. *Am. J. Ophthalmol.* 88:868, 1979.

Kline, L. B., and Glaser, J. S. Dominant optic atrophy. *Arch. Ophthalmol.* 97:1680, 1979.

Lessell, S., and Rosman, N. P. Juvenile diabetes mellitus and optic atrophy. *Arch. Neurol.* 34:759, 1977.

Treft, R. L., et al. Dominant optic atrophy, deafness, ptosis, ophthalmoplegia, dystaxia, and myopathy. *Ophthalmology* 91:908, 1984.

11

Leber's Optic Neuropathy

A 26-year-old man rapidly lost vision in his right eye over a period of 10 days. He had no other symptoms. His history and family history were unremarkable. He received a 3-week course of corticosteroids, but over the next 3-month period vision remained unchanged and he was referred for further evaluation.

Neuro-Ophthalmic Examination

	OD	OS
Visual acuity	20/800	20/20
Color plates correct	None	10 of 10
Pupils	Relative afferent pupillary defect	
Motility, lids, orbits	Normal	Normal
Fundi (see Plate 18)	Hyperemic optic disk	Hyperemic optic disk

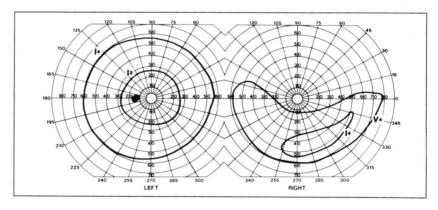

A neurologic examination was normal.

Summary

Three months after rapid visual loss in the right eye, a 26-year-old man was found to have visual acuity of 20/800, a relative afferent pupillary defect, a central scotoma, and disk hyperemia in the right eye. Visual function in the left eye was normal, but the left disk appeared slightly hyperemic.

Differential Diagnosis

The most common cause of sudden monocular visual loss in a young adult is optic neuritis, as described in Chapter 2. However, in at least 85 percent of patients some improvement would have been noted within 3 months of onset. In any male in the teens or twenties with sudden visual loss, particularly in whom there is no improvement within several months, Leber's optic neuropathy must be a consideration. Both eyes are affected in every case but weeks to months may pass before visual loss occurs in the second eye. Although it is an inherited disorder, in some cases of Leber's a history of occurrence in other family members cannot be elicited.

A clue to diagnosis in this case lies in the disk appearance of the left eye. Although the visual field is normal, this disk appears hyperemic and telangiectatic vessels are apparent at the disk margin. This appearance is virtually pathognomonic of Leber's and may be observed before visual loss.

Clinical Diagnosis: Leber's Optic Neuropathy

Described by Leber in 1871, the optic neuropathy that bears his name generally affects males between the ages of 15 and 25. The onset of this disorder has been reported in patients as young as 5 and as old as 65. Visual loss is generally sudden and may progress for days to weeks. Both eyes are involved in virtually all cases although weeks to months may elapse before the second eye is affected. Visual loss is usually severe, with a final visual acuity generally in the range of 20/200 to finger counting. A dense central or cecocentral scotoma is the typical visual field defect.

The optic disk may appear normal or have the pathognomonic appearance of hyperemia, with opacification of the peripapillary nerve fiber layer, which may contain abnormal telangiectatic vessels. The presence of these vessels has suggested a microangiopathy as a pathogenic mechanism. Presymptomatic eyes that will ultimately lose vision and eyes of asymptomatic carriers may show some of these microangiopathic changes and may have disturbances in color vision.

Several months after visual loss, optic atrophy develops and the vascular changes become less prominent. In about 10 percent of cases some recovery of vision, occasionally even to normal, occurs, usually 1 to 2 years after it was lost. The explanation for this is unknown.

In most cases, the optic neuropathy occurs as an isolated event, although a variety of neurologic abnormalities have been reported.

The cause of Leber's disease is unknown. It does not fit into any of the classic mendelian inheritance patterns. It is passed through the female line, with the trait appearing in sons; the carrier state and less commonly the trait also appear in daughters. Males are affected 10 times more commonly than females. The inheritance differs from a sex-linked disorder in that affected males do not pass on the trait or carrier state to their offspring. A variety of causes have been postulated including transplacental or cytoplasmic transfer of a slow virus agent, a mitochondrial inheritance, and a defect in the detoxification of cyanide.

Additional Testing

Fluorescein angiography may be useful to demonstrate better the microangiopathic changes. In addition the angiogram will show that there is no leakage from the disk even when it appears edematous.

If family history of Leber's disease or the pathognomonic funduscopic changes are present, no further workup is necessary. If neither of these features is present, however, it is advisable to evaluate the patient for heavy metal intoxication, nutritional and vitamin deficiencies, compressive lesion (with computed tomography or magnetic resonance imaging [MRI]), and demyelinative disease (MRI, lumbar puncture, evoked potentials).

Management and Course of the Case

Eight months after the loss of vision in the right eye, the patient gradually lost vision over a 3-week period in the left eye to finger counting. The left disk appeared even more hyperemic, and the circumpapillary angiopathy was more apparent than it had been on the initial examination. Fluorescein angiography showed no leakage from the disk.

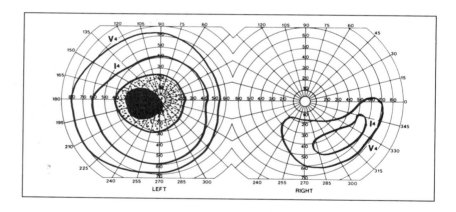

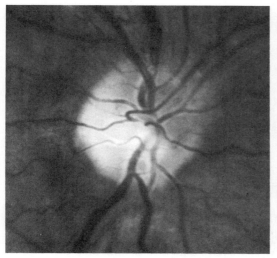 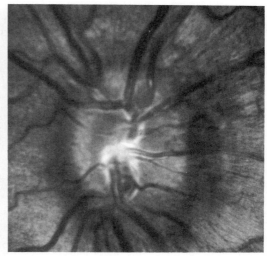

OD   OS

In 2 years of subsequent follow-up the patient's visual function remained unchanged and optic atrophy developed. No other family members were known to have been affected.

Bibliography

Carroll, W. M., and Mastaglia, F. L. Leber's optic neuropathy: A clinical and visual evoked potential study of affected and asymptomatic members of a six generation family. *Brain* 102:559, 1979.

Lessell, S., Gise, R. L., and Krohel, G. B. Bilateral optic neuropathy with remission in young men: Variation on a theme by Leber? *Arch. Neurol.* 40:2, 1983.

Livingstone, R., et al. Leber's optic neuropathy: Clinical and visual evoked response studies in asymptomatic and symptomatic members of a 4-generation family. *Br. J. Ophthalmol.* 64:751, 1980.

Nikoskelainen, E., Hoyt, W. F., and Nummelin, K. Ophthalmoscopic findings in Leber's hereditary optic neuropathy: I. Fundus findings in asymptomatic family members. *Arch. Ophthalmol.* 100:1597, 1982.

Nikoskelainen, E., Hoyt, W. F., and Nummelin, K. The ophthalmoscopic findings in Leber's hereditary optic neuropathy: II. The fundus findings in the affected family members. *Arch. Ophthalmol.* 101:1059, 1983.

Nikoskelainen, E., et al. Fundus findings in Leber's hereditary optic neuroretinopathy: III. Fluorescein angiographic studies. *Arch. Ophthalmol.* 102:981, 1984.

Nikoskelainen, E., et al. The early phase in Leber's hereditary optic atrophy. *Arch. Ophthalmol.* 95:969, 1977.

Smith, J. L., Hoyt, W. F., and Susac, J. O. Ocular fundus in acute Leber's optic neuropathy. *Arch. Ophthalmol.* 90:349, 1973.

Stehouwer, A., et al. Leber's optic neuropathy: II. Fluorescein angiographic studies. *Doc. Ophthalmol.* 53:113, 1982.

Stehouwer, A., and Went, L. N. Leber's optic neuropathy: I. Clinical studies. *Doc. Ophthalmol.* 53:97, 1982.

12

Nutritional Optic Neuropathy

A 56-year-old man developed progressive visual loss in both eyes over a 2-month period.

Neuro-Ophthalmic Examination

	OD	OS
Visual acuity	20/200	20/200
Color plates correct	Control only	Control only
Pupils	Normal	Normal
Motility, lids, orbits	Normal	Normal
Funduscopic appearance	Normal	Normal

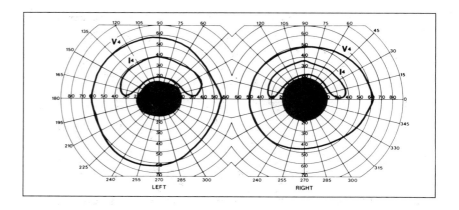

A neurologic examination was normal.

Summary

A 56-year-old man developed a central scotoma and visual acuity of 20/200 in each eye over a 2-month period. His optic disk and retina in each eye appeared normal.

Differential Diagnosis

The most common causes of bilateral central scotomas that develop gradually include nutritional optic neuropathy, tobacco-alcohol amblyopia, vitamin B$_{12}$ and folate deficiency, drug toxicity (e.g., chloramphenicol, ethambutol, chlorpropamide, ethchlorvynol [Placidyl]), heavy metal or methanol poisoning, hereditary optic atrophy, and infiltrative disorders (carcinomatous, lymphoreticular, or granulomatous—sarcoidosis, syphilis, tuberculosis). Less common causes include a compressive lesion (although possible; see Bilateral Central Scotomas from Meningioma, below), bilateral optic neuritis, and a retinal cone dystrophy (see Cone Dystrophy, below).

A detailed medical, social, drug, diet, work, and family history is key to diagnosis in these cases.

Additional History

The patient admitted that he had been an alcohol abuser for the past 25 years. For several months before the onset of visual loss he had been imbibing heavily and his diet had consisted mainly of carbohydrates. He had also been a one-pack-per-day cigarette smoker for 30 years.

Clinical Diagnosis: Nutritional Optic Neuropathy (Tobacco-Alcohol Amblyopia)

The cause of tobacco-alcohol amblyopia remains controversial. Whether it is the result of a toxic effect of alcohol or tobacco or both or due to an associated vitamin deficiency is unknown. Since most affected patients drink alcohol, smoke cigarettes, and have a substandard diet, it is difficult to separate the various potential causative factors. In patients who are heavy tobacco users, cyanide toxicity has been postulated as the mechanism.

Visual loss in this disorder varies from mild to severe. It is always bilateral, although involvement of the two eyes may be asymmetric. There is selective involvement of the papillomacular bundle, and thus a central or cecocentral scotoma is generally present but the peripheral field is normal. Visual acuity is often decreased to 20/200.

At the time of presentation the optic disks generally appear normal. Splinter hemorrhages and tortuosity of small retinal vessels in the posterior pole may be present. Later, optic disk pallor may develop.

If the treatment regimen outlined below is followed, the chances of visual recovery over a period of several months are good. However, if alcohol and tobacco use and poor nutrition continue, the loss may be permanent.

Additional Testing

A blood count, serum vitamin B$_{12}$ and folate levels, VDRL test, and chest x-rays should be performed in all cases unless a specific diagnosis is apparent. When a nutritional cause is not suspected, a heavy metal screen, lumbar puncture, and computed tomography (CT) should be performed. If the diagnosis still remains unknown, further workup for demyelinative disease or systemic infiltrative disorders may be indicated.

Treatment

Treatment of a nutritional optic neuropathy (tobacco-alcohol amblyopia) should consist of a cessation of both alcohol and tobacco use, a well-balanced diet, and B complex vitamins. Treatment with hydroxycobalamin, 1000 mg intramuscularly once a month, may be considered.

Management and Course of the Case

The patient entered an alcohol rehabilitation program and ceased cigarette smoking. He took B complex vitamins daily and received an intramuscular injection of hydroxycobalamin, 1000 mg monthly. After 3 months his vision began to improve, and after 9 months visual acuity was 20/50 in the right eye and 20/60 in the left eye. There was no further improvement in 2 years of follow-up.

Cone Dystrophy

A 28-year-old man who gradually lost vision in both eyes over several years beginning at about age 17 was found in each eye to have visual acuity of 20/100, a marked dyschromatopsia (he identified the control color plate only), a central scotoma, mild temporal disk pallor, and an abnormal-appearing macula. A fluorescein angiogram demonstrated a macular disturbance. The right eye is pictured on p. 95. Funduscopic appearance and fluorescein angiography were identical in the left eye.

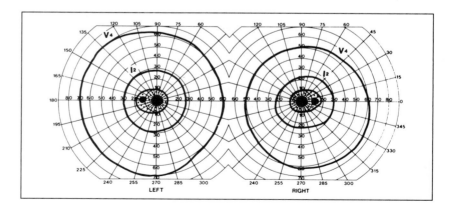

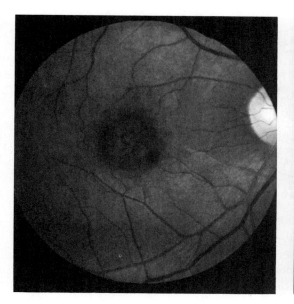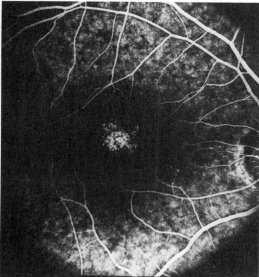

A diagnosis of cone dystrophy was established on electroretinography, which showed an absent photopic response and mildly abnormal scotopic response.

Progressive cone-rod dystrophy is an inherited condition affecting both eyes, with visual loss usually beginning in the teens and worsening over several years. Inheritance is most commonly autosomal dominant. Early in the disease, funduscopic and electrophysiologic changes may be minimal, making definitive diagnosis impossible. Later the diagnosis becomes more obvious.

Bilateral Central Scotomas from Meningioma

A 46-year-old woman who gradually lost vision in both eyes over a 6-month period was found to have visual acuity of 20/50 in the right eye and 20/800 in the left, dyschromatopsia in both eyes (she identified one color plate OD, none OS), and a central scotoma in the visual field in each eye. Funduscopic appearance was normal.

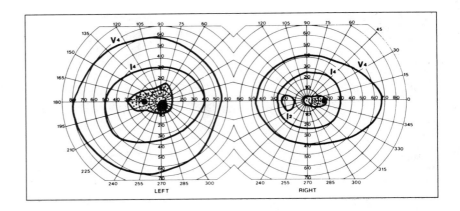

There was no history of alcohol or tobacco use, drug or toxin exposure, or family members with visual loss, and her nutrition was good. Results of her initial blood workup were normal. A CT scan showed a large mass, which at craniotomy was found to be a meningioma.

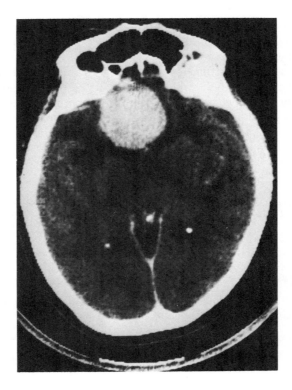

This case represents an extremely rare occurrence of an intracranial compressive lesion producing central scotomas without loss of peripheral field and without evidence of chiasmal involvement. Although the progressive onset of central scotomas usually has a nutritional, toxic, or hereditary cause, when a cause is not determined CT or magnetic resonance imaging should be performed to rule out a compressive lesion.

Bibliography

Carroll, F. D. Etiology and treatment of tobacco-alcohol amblyopia. *Am. J. Ophthalmol.* 27:713, 1944.

Foulds, W. S., Chisholm, I. A., and Pettigrew, A. R. The toxic optic neuropathies. *Br. J. Ophthalmol.* 58:386, 1974.

Frisen, L. Fundus changes in acute malnutritional optic neuropathy. *Arch. Ophthalmol.* 101:577, 1983.

Kupersmith, M. J., Weiss, P. A., and Carr, R. E. The visual-evoked potential in tobacco-alcohol and nutritional amblyopia. *Am. J. Ophthalmol.* 95:307, 1983.

Page, N. G. R., and Sanders, M. D. Bilateral central scotomata due to intracranial tumour. *Br. J. Ophthalmol.* 68:449, 1984.

Potts, A. M. Tobacco amblyopia. *Surv. Ophthalmol.* 17:313, 1973.

13

Traumatic Optic Neuropathy

In a motor vehicle accident, a 32-year-old man struck the right frontal area of his head and lost consciousness for 2 hours. On awakening he noted that his vision was reduced in the right eye. Skull and optic canal x-rays and computed tomography scans were normal. At the time of his evaluation the next day, there had been no change in his vision from the time of the accident.

Neuro-Ophthalmic Examination

	OD	OS
Visual acuity	20/400	20/20
Pupils	Relative afferent pupillary defect	
Motility, lids, orbits	Normal	Normal
Funduscopic appearance	Normal	Normal

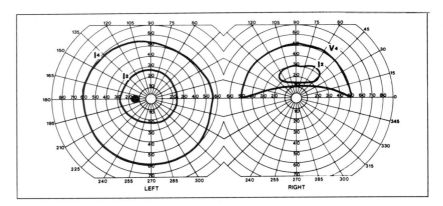

A neurologic examination was normal.

Summary
A 32-year-old man who suffered visual loss in the right eye from a head injury had visual acuity of 20/400, a relative afferent pupillary defect, marked loss of visual field, and a normal-appearing optic disk and retina in the right eye.

Differential Diagnosis

The presence of a relative afferent pupillary defect with unilateral visual field loss and normal funduscopic appearance localizes the damage to the right optic nerve. The presumption must be that the visual loss occurred from the accident and was not preexisting. If optic atrophy had been present on the initial examination, a preexisting abnormality would have had to have been present.

Clinical Diagnosis: Traumatic Optic Neuropathy

Damage to the optic nerve occurs in about 5 percent of head injuries. The blow is typically to the ipsilateral frontal area and usually is severe enough to produce loss of consciousness. Most of the injuries to the nerve occur within the optic canal where the nerve is immobilized by the firm attachment of its dural sheath to the bony wall. A likely mechanism for nerve damage is the production of shearing forces that, when induced in the immobile nerve by the movement of the brain in an anterior-posterior direction from the frontal impact, could either damage the nerve fibers directly or disrupt their blood supply. Edema or hemorrhage can also be factors by compressing the nerve within the optic canal. A fracture of the canal can be radiographically demonstrated in fewer than one-third of cases. Blunt trauma only rarely injures the optic nerve within the orbit where the nerve has considerable slack.

Optic nerve injuries are almost always unilateral. Visual loss can range from mild—just a visual field defect with no reduction in visual acuity—to severe (no light perception). Unless the optic nerve is damaged within the orbit (in which case a picture of central retinal artery occlusion may be present), the optic disk and retina will initially appear normal. Diagnosis is established based on the presence of a relative afferent pupillary defect and unilateral visual loss.

Additional Testing

Computed tomography should be performed to evaluate for a fracture of the canal and for the presence of hemorrhage.

Treatment and Prognosis

In most cases visual loss is at a maximum from the time of impact and shows no meaningful improvement. No treatment has been proved to be of value. The Japanese literature cites an extremely high success rate with optic canal decompression, but this has not been the experience in the United States. Megadose corticosteroids (dexamethasone 3–5 mg/kg/day) have been reported to be effective in some cases. We consider this therapy in some patients without a systemic contraindication seen within 24 hours of the injury, but if there is no improvement within 48 hours would discontinue it. Should improvement occur we would switch to oral therapy and taper over about two weeks. If vision regresses during the taper, we would then consider decompression of the optic canal.

In a minority of cases, visual loss is delayed or progressive, presumably from edema of the nerve or hemorrhage within the canal. All such documented cases should be considered for either megadose corticosteroid therapy or optic canal decompression through either a transethmoidal or transfrontal approach. If the steroid option is chosen and visual function does not improve within 8 to 12 hours, or if vision improves but then worsens as steroids are tapered, decompression is indicated.

In the typical case in which no improvement in vision occurs, optic disk pallor will first appear between 3 and 4 weeks after the injury.

Management and Course of the Case

Since visual loss appeared to be from the time of impact, no treatment for the optic neuropathy was instituted. There was no change in the patient's visual function in 1 year of follow-up. The right disk became pale.

Traumatic Chiasmal Syndrome

In a motor vehicle accident a 19-year-old man suffered a severe frontal blow that produced a skull fracture and loss of consciousness for 2 weeks. He was found to have a bitemporal visual field defect and later was diagnosed to have diabetes insipidus.

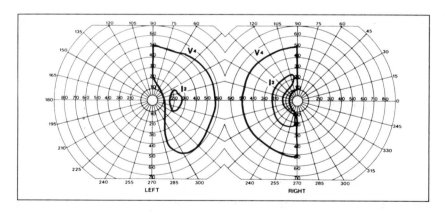

Optic chiasmal damage occurs much less commonly than optic nerve damage in blunt head injuries. The blow is usually frontal and severe. Visual loss generally does not improve.

Traumatic retrochiasmal involvement producing a homonymous hemianopia is also uncommon.

Bibliography

Anderson, R. L., Panje, W. R., and Gross, C. E. Optic nerve blindness following blunt forehead trauma. *Ophthalmology* 89:445, 1982.

Fukado, Y. Results in 400 cases of surgical decompression of the optic nerve. *Mod. Probl. Ophthalmol.* 14:474, 1975.

Imachi, J., Inoue, K., and Takahashi, T. Clinical and pathohistological investigations of optic nerve lesions in cases of head injuries. *Jpn. J. Ophthalmol.* 12:20, 1968.

Kline, L. B., Morawetz, R. B., and Swaid, S. N. Indirect injury of the optic nerve. *Neurosurgery* 14:756, 1984.

Savino, P. J., Glaser, J. S., and Schatz, N. J. Traumatic chiasmal syndrome. *Neurology* 30:963, 1980.

14

Optic Nerve Hypoplasia

A 9-month-old boy was evaluated becaue of poor vision and nystagmus. He had been the product of an uncomplicated term pregnancy; his birth weight had been 7 lb, 1 oz. Other than visually, growth and development had been normal.

Neuro-Ophthalmic Examination

	OU
Visual acuity	Poor fixation and following
Pupils	Sluggish
Motility	Full range of movement
	Horizontal pendular nystagmus
Fundi	Optic nerve hypoplasia

The fundus of the left eye is shown in Plate 19. The right eye appeared similar.

A neurologic examination was normal.

Summary

A 9-month-old infant with poor vision and nystagmus was found to have abnormal optic disks.

Clinical Diagnosis: Optic Nerve Hypoplasia

Optic nerve hypoplasia is a developmental anomaly of unknown causation. Although there is an association with maternal ingestion of quinine, LSD, anticonvulsants, and other medications as well as maternal diabetes mellitus, in most cases a causal factor cannot be identified. Familial cases are extremely rare. The defect may be unilateral or bilateral and may be an isolated finding or associated with other anomalies.

Diagnosis is established on ophthalmoscopy by the appearance of the disk, which appears small. The nerve tissue may occupy the center of the disk or may be at the disk rim with a large central excavation. A double ring of pigmentation, which represents the junction between the sclera and lamina cribrosa (outer ring) and the termination of the retinal pigment epithelium (inner ring), may surround the disk. In some cases the edge of the small disk may blend in with the circumpapillary tissue, and only with careful ophthalmoscopy can the hypoplastic nature of the disk be identified.

The level of visual acuity varies. In cases of severe hypoplasia vision is very poor, but with lesser degrees vision may be good. Occasionally visual acuity may be normal with only a visual field defect present. When the anomaly is bilateral and severe, nystagmus is usually present.

Bilateral cases are much more likely to be associated with other anomalies than unilateral cases. Associated ocular abnormalities include microphthalmos and uveal, retinal, and optic nerve colobomas. Abnormalities may be found in anterior midline structures of the brain or cranium—maldevelopment of the optic chiasm, absence of the septum pellucidum, pituitary dysfunction, agenesis of the corpus callosum, basal encephaloceles, hypertelorism, and others. There also may be associated anomalies of the brain such as areas of porencephaly, and developmental delay may occur. De Morsier described the septo-optic dysplasia syndrome as consisting of optic nerve hypoplasia, nystagmus, absence of the septum pellucidum, and short stature (from hypopituitarism).

Plate 20 shows another type of congenital optic nerve anomaly: optic disk coloboma.

Additional Testing

The extent of the systemic evaluation for associated anomalies must be individualized. If the child appears to be a normal healthy infant in whom growth rate and development are normal for his or her age, observation without additional testing is reasonable. However, if growth is retarded or development in any area is slow, a neurologic and endocrinologic evaluation is advisable including neuroradiologic scanning and pituitary function studies.

Management and Course of the Case

The patient was examined for related anomalies because of the bilateral severe nature of the optic nerve hypoplasia. Computed tomography and pituitary function test results were normal.

The Infant with Poor Vision: Differential Diagnosis

When asked to examine an infant with reduced vision in whom the diagnosis is not obvious (i.e., no apparent ocular cause) one should consider several conditions. As mentioned above the diagnosis of optic nerve hypoplasia is not always obvious, and careful ophthalmoscopy is necessary to rule this out as a possibility.

DEVELOPMENTAL DELAY

Poor fixational ability in an infant could be related to slow development. An infant will normally fix on and follow a target by 3 months of age, but in some infants this is delayed. Although occasionally a delay in visual development will occur for several months in an otherwise normal infant, more often the child's overall development is slow and vision is just a part of the whole picture. If a child reaches a sixth-month level of development and still does not appear to see, an investigation for a cause is warranted.

CORTICAL BLINDNESS
Damage to the geniculocalcarine pathway bilaterally owing either to maldevelopment (e.g., porencephaly) or to anoxia would impair vision. Almost always, visual impairment would not be an isolated neurologic finding. Thus, in a child who is developing normally, this is an unlikely diagnosis.

RETINAL DISORDERS
In certain inherited retinal conditions, there may be no or minimal funduscopic findings and additional testing is necessary for diagnosis.

Congenital Achromatopsia. In congenital achromatopsia, an autosomal recessively inherited condition, there is a congenital absence or reduction in the number of cones in the retina. In the typical case visual acuity is reduced to the level of 20/200, color vision is markedly abnormal, and nystagmus and photophobia are present. A paradoxical pupillary response with dilation in light and constriction when light is removed has been described. There are often no perceptible funduscopic changes, but a reduction in the foveal reflex or a mild retinal pigment epithelial disturbance may be present. Fluorescein angiography may be normal or show mild retinal pigment epithelial changes. Diagnosis is established on electroretinography: The photopic response is absent or markedly reduced, while the scotopic response is relatively normal. Visual loss tends not to be progressive. The photophobia and nystagmus tend to lessen in the teenage years.

Leber's Congenital Amaurosis. Not to be confused with Leber's hereditary optic neuropathy, Leber's congenital amaurosis, an autosomal recessively inherited condition, is a generalized retinal degeneration that begins at or shortly after birth. In most cases visual loss is severe (in the range of 20/200 to hand motion), and nystagmus or searching eye movements are present. The funduscopic picture varies from normal to that of tapetoretinal degeneration with diffuse retinal pigmentary changes, narrowed arterioles, and disk pallor. In many cases in which the retina initially appears normal, pigmentary changes later appear. Diagnosis is established by the electroretinogram, which will be flat or show only minimal response.

Albinism. Albinism may occur with (oculocutaneous) or without (ocular) obvious abnormalities in skin pigmentation. Ocular albinism is inherited in an X-linked recessive or autosomal recessive pattern. Vision is decreased relative to the amount of reduction in pigmentation. In severe cases visual acuity is reduced to 20/400 or worse. Diagnosis is established by the recognition of foveal hypoplasia and transillumination defects in the iris, although the latter may not be appreciated in blacks. The hair bulb incubation test for tyrosinase performed on a skin biopsy specimen will have a positive result. An electroretinogram will show a normal or supernormal response. A characteristic visually evoked potential response may be present.

Bibliography

Margalith, D., et al. Clinical spectrum of congenital optic nerve hypoplasia: Review of 51 patients. *Dev. Med. Child. Neurol.* 26:311, 1984.

Nelson, M., Lessell, S., and Sadun, A. A. Optic nerve hypoplasia and maternal diabetes mellitus. *Arch. Neurol.* 43:20, 1986.

Skarf, B., and Hoyt, C. S. Optic nerve hypoplasia in children: Association with anomalies of the endocrine and cns. *Arch. Ophthalmol.* 102:62, 1984.

Wilson, D. M., et al. Computed tomographic findings in septo-optic dysplasia: Discordance between clinical and radiological findings. *Neuroradiology* 26:279, 1984.

15

Amaurosis Fugax

A 60-year-old man was examined because of an episode of visual loss in the left eye 2 days earlier that had lasted 15 minutes. Six months earlier he had experienced a similar episode in the left eye. He had not experienced any transient cerebrovascular symptoms. He had suffered a myocardial infarction 2 years earlier but appeared to be in good general health. There was no history of migraine. He was taking no medications.

The results of a neuro-ophthalmic examination, a neurologic examination, and carotid and cardiac auscultation were normal.

Summary

A 60-year-old man who suffered two episodes of transient visual loss in the left eye appeared normal on examination.

Differential Diagnosis

There are a number of causes of transient visual loss. The description of the episode, the presence of any associated symptoms, and the patient's history would help limit the number of possible diagnoses. The conditions that most commonly produce visual loss of the duration in this case include emboli from the carotid or heart, hypoperfusion secondary to carotid stenosis, and migraine. Other conditions—vasculitis (giant cell arteritis in the elderly, systemic lupus erythematosus in younger patients), increased intracranial pressure, anemia, hypotension, myopia, disk drusen—may be associated with transient visual symptoms but they are usually of short duration and would not be a major consideration in this case. However, it is important to emphasize that in patients over 60 years old, giant cell arteritis should always be given some thought. Uhthoff's phenomena—temporary visual loss occurring with overheating after optic nerve demyelination—is an occasional diagnostic consideration. Transient occipital ischemia must also be considered. Although it produces a homonymous deficit in both eyes, patients will frequently attribute the visual loss to just the eye on the side of the affected field. Careful questioning of the patient in regard to how vision was impaired is thus necessary.

In the present case of a 60-year-old man, carotid disease is the most likely cause. A cardiac source for emboli would be much less likely. Migraine could produce identical visual symptoms but in a patient this age without a history of migraine, it can only be considered a diagnosis of exclusion. The patient had no symptoms suggestive of giant cell arteritis.

Clinical Diagnosis: Amaurosis Fugax Secondary to Carotid Disease

As mentioned above, visual loss can occur from either emboli or high-grade carotid stenosis. In the former circumstance visual loss typically lasts from 5 to 30 minutes, whereas in the latter it may be shorter. The patient may describe the episode in a number of ways. A curtain dropping over the eye is a classic description, but more often the patient will just note a blackout or "grayout" of all or part of the vision or just blurring of vision. Recognition of a plaque in a retinal arteriole or a carotid bruit is important in diagnosis, but in many cases neither is present. With each episode of amaurosis, a permanent visual deficit is possible although the incidence is low.

Additional Testing

A general physical examination with attention to the cardiovascular system should be performed. Blood studies should include glucose, cholesterol, and triglyceride levels and an erythrocyte sedimentation rate.

What type of carotid artery evaluation to perform is controversial. Since it is usually already presumed that the patient has carotid disease, noninvasive studies that may screen for this have a limited role in decision making. In a reliable laboratory, noninvasive tests may be of value in following the progression of carotid disease. Digital venous subtraction angiography has not proved to be a useful test since it generally does not obviate the need for arteriography. The major decision that must be made in cases of amaurosis fugax is whether endarterectomy is to be considered. If so, arteriography must be performed. Digital arteriography may be considered.

Treatment

The risk of visual loss or stroke in a patient with amaurosis fugax has not been well studied but probably is on the order of about 5 percent per year. A treatment that would lower this risk without serious morbidity would be worthwhile. Both medical and surgical therapies have a role.

Medical treatment generally consists of antiplatelet drugs, with aspirin being the most popular agent. The proper dosage of aspirin is not established. Dipyridamole (Persantine) in a dosage of 50 mg three times daily is an alternate choice. Antiplatelet drugs have been shown to reduce the incidence of stroke in patients with transient ischemic attacks and thus presumably would do so in amaurosis fugax. More important, these medications reduce the incidence of myocardial infarction, which occurs with a high frequency in patients with amaurosis fugax as well as transient ischemic attacks. The death rate from myocardial infarction is much higher than the death rate from stroke in patients with amaurosis fugax or transient ischemic attacks. Anticoagulation with heparin or warfarin sodium (Coumadin) is of value when there is a cardiac source of emboli but is generally not prescribed for amaurosis fugax occurring in isolation secondary to carotid disease. In an exceptional patient with very frequent episodes of amaurosis fugax this treatment might be considered.

Endarterectomy also reduces the incidence of stroke in patients with transient ischemic attacks. The morbidity and mortality of the procedure vary considerably with the expertise of the surgeon but are optimally 1 to 2 percent.

Unfortunately antiplatelet therapy and endarterectomy have not been compared in patients either with amaurosis fugax or transient ischemic attacks in a controlled clinical trial. The decision on which treatment to advise must be individualized. Factors favoring commencement with aspirin include infrequent episodes, particularly if more than a month has passed since the last one; no cerebrovascular symptoms; previous myocardial infarction, serious systemic vascular disease, or other systemic disease that might complicate surgery; lack of a highly skilled surgeon; and the patient's desire to avoid surgery. Factors favoring an evaluation for endarterectomy include multiple episodes of amaurosis fugax, particularly if recent; occurrence of transient ischemic attacks; good general health; availability of a skilled, experienced surgeon; and the occurrence of attacks during antiplatelet therapy.

Management and Course of the Case
The clinician recommended arteriography and consideration for endarterectomy. However, the patient did not wish to have surgery. Therapy with 60 mg of aspirin per day was begun. In 2 years of follow-up he has remained asymptomatic.

Transient Visual Loss in a Young Adult

A 20-year-old woman who was examined because of one episode of a blackout of vision in the right eye for 15 minutes was otherwise asymptomatic, and results of a neuro-ophthalmic and neurologic examination were normal. She had suffered throbbing holocranial headaches associated with nausea about six times a year since age 15. Retinal migraine was presumed to be the cause of the visual symptoms.

In a young person transient monocular visual loss is usually attributed to migraine, even when there is not a clear-cut history of vascular headaches. Visual loss generally lasts 5 to 30 minutes. Headache may or may not accompany the visual loss. With a strong history of migraine, it can be presumed to be the diagnosis. Without such a history the patient should undergo a general physical examination, and a blood count and antinuclear antibody determination should be obtained. An echocardiogram may be considered. Carotid studies are not performed routinely but should be reserved for the atypical patient with recurrent episodes despite therapy or with associated neurologic symptoms.

If the episodes are infrequent, observation without therapy is warranted. Birth control pills should be discontinued. If the episodes are occurring with some frequency, however, migraine prophylactic treatment should be prescribed. Low-dose aspirin alone is sometimes of value. If not, a beta blocker should be considered.

Hollenhorst Plaque

On routine examination a 72-year-old man was found to have a plaque in a retinal arteriole in his right eye. His examination results were normal.

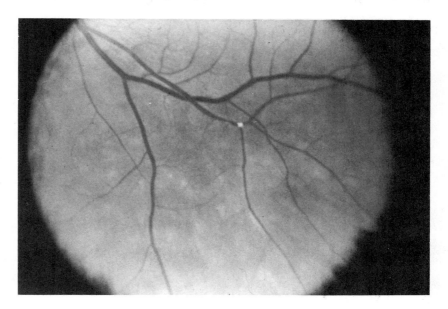

The workup and treatment of a patient with an asymptomatic retinal plaque is controversial. Since generally it is not possible to determine whether the embolus was recent, it is reasonable to consider an asymptomatic patient the same as a patient who has suffered a single episode of amaurosis fugax. The decision as to whether to start antiplatelet therapy or consider arteriography and endarterectomy must be individualized.

Bibliography
Adams, H. P., et al. Amaurosis fugax: The results of arteriography in 59 patients. *Stroke* 14:742, 1983.
Beck, R. W. Amaurosis fugax—controversies in management. *Int. Ophthalmol. Clin.* 26(4):277, 1986.

Canadian Cooperative Study Group. A randomized trial of aspirin and sulfin-pyrazone in threatened stroke. *N. Engl. J. Med.* 299:53, 1978.

Fields, et al. Joint study of extracranial arterial occlusion: V. Progress report of prognosis following surgery or nonsurgical treatment for transient cerebral ischemic attacks and cervical cartoid artery lesions. *J.A.M.A.* 211:1993, 1970.

Fisher, C. M. Late-life migraine accompaniments as a cause of unexplained transient ischemic attacks. *Can. J. Neurol. Sci.* 7:9, 1980.

Hooshmand, H., et al. Amaurosis fugax: Diagnostic and therapeutic aspects. *Stroke* 5:643, 1974.

Hurwitz, B. J., et al. Comparison of amaurosis and transient cerebral ischemia: A prospective clinical and arteriographic study. *Ann. Neurol.* 18:698, 1985.

Kistler, J. P., Ropper, A. H., and Heros, R. C. Therapy of ischemic cerebral vascular disease due to atherothrombosis (part 1). *N. Engl. J. Med.* 311:27, 1984.

Kistler, J. P., Ropper, A. H., and Heros, R. C. Therapy of ischemic cerebral vascular disease due to atherothrombosis (part 2). *N. Engl. J. Med.* 311:100, 1984.

Lieppman, M. E. Intermittent visual "white out": A new intraocular lens complication. *Ophthalmology* 89:109, 1982.

Marshall, J., and Meadows, S. The natural history of amaurosis fugax. *Brain* 91:419, 1968.

Mungas, J. E., and Baker, W. H. Amaurosis fugax. *Stroke* 8:232, 1977.

Parkin, P. J., et al. Amaurosis fugax: Some aspects of management. *J. Neurol. Neurosurg. Psychiatry* 45:1, 1982.

Poole, C. J. M., and Russell, R. W. R. Mortality and stroke after amaurosis fugax. *J. Neurol. Neurosurg. Psychiatry* 48:902, 1985.

Savino, P. J., Glaser, J. S., and Cassady, J. Retinal stroke: Is the patient at risk? *Arch. Ophthalmol.* 95:1185, 1977.

Trobe, J. D. Carotid endarterectomy. Who needs it? *Ophthalmology* 94:725, 1987.

16

Uncommon Optic Neuropathies

Papillophlebitis

A 23-year-old woman who noted mild blurring of vision in the right eye was found to have visual acuity of 20/20 in both eyes, swelling of the right optic disk (see Plate 21), and an enlarged blind spot in the right eye on perimetry. The left disk and field were normal.

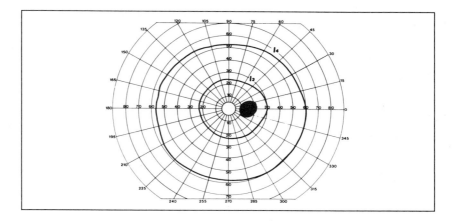

A computed tomography (CT) scan was normal. A diagnosis of papillophlebitis was made. The patient was treated with corticosteroids for 1 month, with resolution of the disk edema over a 2-month period.

Papillophlebitis is an ill-defined entity characterized by unilateral optic disk swelling, usually in young adults. Optic nerve function is generally normal, and perimetry typically shows only enlargement of the blind spot. The optic disk swelling can be quite marked. Scattered retinal hemorrhages are also occasionally seen. Diagnosis is a clinical one. CT to rule out a compressive lesion may be prudent, although it would be extremely unusual for such a lesion to produce disk edema without loss of vision. The cause of papillophlebitis is unknown; inflammation of the central retinal vein has been postulated. The course is usually benign, with no loss of vision and resolution of the disk edema over several months. Whether corticosteroid therapy is beneficial is not known.

A 55-year-old asymptomatic woman was noted on routine examination to have swelling of the left disk. She had a history of controlled hypertension. Visual acuity was 20/20 in each eye. The left optic disk was hyperemic and swollen. Retinal veins were dilated and there were a few scattered retinal hemorrhages in the periphery (see Plate 22). The right eye was normal. Results of perimetry are shown below.

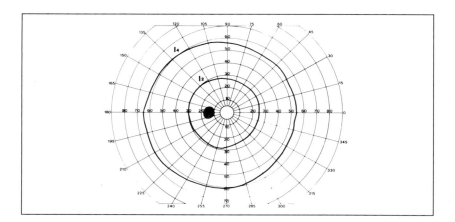

This case represents a syndrome similar to the so-called papillophlebitis. Disk swelling occurs with preserved optic nerve function. The dilation of the retinal veins and the retinal hemorrhages that are often seen suggest that the cause is a partial central retinal vein occlusion or a complete occlusion with good collateral venous flow. Progression to a full-blown central retinal vein occlusion is uncommon. The disk edema tends to persist and optociliary shunt vessels may form, but visual function generally remains normal.

Diabetic Papillopathy

A 17-year-old diabetic girl developed blurred vision in both eyes over a period of 2 weeks. Vision was 20/20 in the right eye and 20/25 in the left, but there was marked loss of visual field in both eyes. Both optic disks were swollen, with prominent telangiectatic vessels overlying the disk surface (see Plate 23).

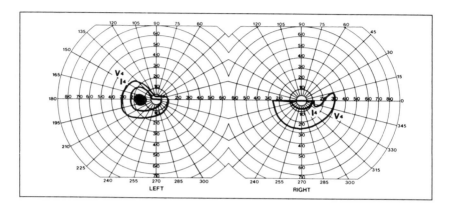

A CT scan and lumbar puncture results were normal. A diagnosis of diabetic papillopathy was made. Disk edema resolved over a 3-month period, but the visual field deficits remained.

This case represents an uncommon condition in which disk edema occurs in association with juvenile diabetes mellitus. Involvement can be unilateral or bilateral. Onset is typically insidious, and the disk edema may be an incidental finding in an asymptomatic patient. Visual field defects as extensive as those in this case are uncommon. More typically the field deficits are minimal, and enlargement of the blind spot may be the only abnormality. The presence of telangiectatic vessels overlying the swollen disk is particularly characteristic of this entity, and recognition of this is useful in diagnosis. When the condition is unilateral, a clinical diagnosis can be made without additional testing. When it is bilateral, it may be necessary to rule out increased intracranial pressure. Disk edema generally resolves over several months. Visual field defects tend to remain permanently. No treatment is known to be of value.

The cause of this condition is unknown. It tends to affect insulin-dependent diabetics in their teens and twenties. There does not appear to be any relationship to the degree of diabetic control or presence of diabetic retinopathy. The condition differs from the routine ischemic optic neuropathy in that involvement is often simultaneously bilateral and optic nerve function is often not impaired.

Thyroid Optic Neuropathy

A 51-year-old woman gradually lost vision in the right eye over a 2-month period. She also had experienced intermittent diplopia for 4 months. She had been diagnosed as having hyperthyroidism 4 years earlier and had been treated with radioactive iodine. Visual acuity was 20/200 in the right eye and 20/20 in the left. A right relative afferent pupillary defect was present. Both optic disks appeared normal. The left visual field was normal. The right field is presented below.

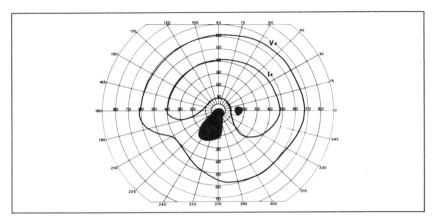

CT demonstrated enlarged extraocular muscles, more so in the right than the left orbit.

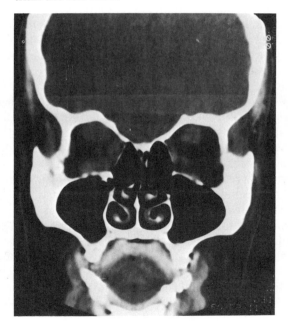

A diagnosis of compressive optic neuropathy from Graves' disease was made, and an orbital decompression was performed. Within 4 weeks vision improved to 20/20 with a full field.

With CT, the optic neuropathy of Graves' disease has been shown to be due to compression of the nerve at the orbital apex by the enlarged muscles. Visual loss tends to be gradual, although a rapid deterioration is possible. There is no relationship between the degree of proptosis and the development of the optic neuropathy. In some patients no proptosis is apparent. The optic disk may appear normal, pale, or swollen at the time of presentation.

In most cases treatment is indicated to prevent progressive visual loss. If visual loss is mild (20/30 or better acuity with minimal field loss), it is reasonable to follow the patient, providing frequent observation is possible. When visual loss is greater, treatment with systemic corticosteroids, orbital decompressive surgery, or orbital radiation is warranted. The decision on which modality to employ must be individualized. With early intervention the prognosis for visual recovery is good.

When visual loss is not severe and there are no systemic contraindications, corticosteroid therapy may be considered. Dosages of 60 to 100 mg per day of prednisone are usually prescribed. If there is no improvement within 1 to 2 weeks, this therapy is not likely to be of benefit and the medication should be tapered. If meaningful improvement does occur, then the corticosteroids should be continued at a moderately high dose for several weeks and then slowly tapered with careful monitoring of visual function. Unfortunately, a large percentage of patients who have a good response will have a flare of the disease as the steroids are reduced. If this occurs, the dosage can be increased and then tapered more slowly. Should the disease flare again, it is advisable to seek another modality of therapy.

In cases with severe visual loss or with a contraindication to or failure of corticosteroids, a surgical decompression should be considered. Orbital radiation (2000 rad in 10 fractions over a 2-week period) is an alternative therapy, particularly in the patient in whom surgery may be risky.

Sarcoid Optic Neuropathy

A 30-year-old man who had had known pulmonary sarcoidosis for 4 years rapidly lost vision in the left eye to light perception. The left disk was swollen (see Plate 24). The right disk was normal. A diagnosis of sarcoid optic neuropathy was made.

Infiltration of the optic nerve with granulomatous inflammation is a possible sequela of sarcoidosis. The disk may have a characteristic white, lumpy, swollen appearance. The degree of visual loss varies considerably from no loss of optic nerve function to severe loss. Most cases are responsive to corticosteroids. Optic nerve involvement in sarcoidosis may be associated with either ocular or central nervous system involvement or may appear to be an isolated finding. Chiasmal involvement is also possible, and sarcoidosis is always in the differential diagnosis of parachiasmal lesions.

Optic Disk Infarct—6:45 Syndrome

A 70-year-old asymptomatic woman was found to have a superior arcuate field defect associated with cupping to the inferior temporal rim in the left eye. In the right eye there was a hemorrhage at the inferior temporal edge of the disk but a normal field (see Plate 25). Acuity was normal in both eyes.

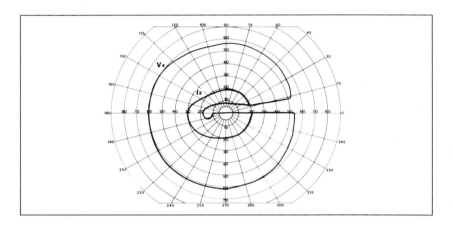

The pistol-like visual field defect in the left eye associated with focal disk cupping appears to be an entity distinct from either glaucoma or anterior ischemic optic neuropathy. It has been called optic disk infarct or the 6:45 syndrome, because of the location of the disk cupping in the right eye between the 6 and 7 o'clock locations at the edge of the disk. The cause is unknown. The defects are generally nonprogressive and not associated with an increase in intraocular pressure. They are often bilateral.

In this case the patient ultimately developed cupping at the location of the hemorrhage in the right eye, and a superior pistollike visual field defect, similar to the defect in the left eye, developed.

Shock Optic Neuropathy

A 67-year-old woman was hospitalized because of a bleeding gastric ulcer. She became hypotensive and required a transfusion of 5 units of blood. At that time she also noted blurred vision in both eyes. On examination 5 days later visual acuity was 20/20 in each eye. Inferior field defects (see below) and mild disk edema were present bilaterally (see Plate 26).

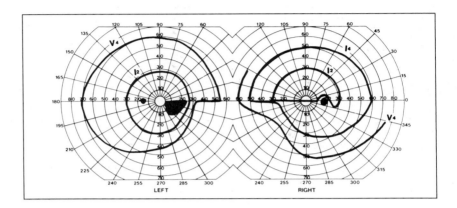

A diagnosis of shock-induced optic neuropathy was made. The edema resolved over a 2-week period, but the field defects persisted.

The optic neuropathy from shock resembles ischemic optic neuropathy in that optic disk edema is associated with nerve fiber bundle visual field defects. Disk hemorrhage is sometimes more prominent than edema. Visual loss is generally permanent. Cupping of the disk may occur, mimicking glaucoma.

Syphilis

A 45-year-old man developed blurred vision in both eyes over several days. In the preceding several months he had suffered headaches, arthralgias, tinnitus, weight loss, alopecia, and intermittent visual blurring. Visual acuity was 20/60 in the right eye and 20/50 in the left with visual field deficits in both eyes (see below). Both optic disks were swollen with moderate vitreous reaction (see Plate 27).

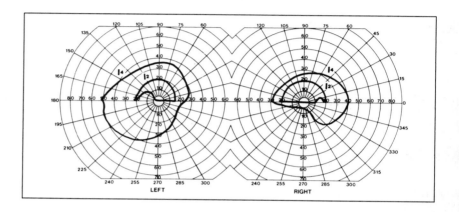

On lumbar puncture there were 59 white blood cells, a protein level of 71 mg/dl, and a positive VDRL test result at a titer of 1 : 8. A diagnosis of syphilis was made, and the patient was treated with penicillin intravenously. Vision improved to 20/20 in each eye over a period of several months.

Optic nerve involvement in syphilis may take several forms. An acute optic neuritis may occur in secondary syphilis as in this case. Optic disk swelling may also occur as part of an ocular inflammatory syndrome from syphilis. Tertiary syphilis can produce a primary optic atrophy. Diagnosis of syphilitic optic neuritis can usually be made on cerebrospinal fluid examination by finding a positive VDRL titer.

Radiation Optic Neuropathy

A 72-year-old woman rapidly lost vision in the right eye. Sixteen months earlier she had had a pituitary tumor surgically removed and received 4500 rad to the sellar area. Visual fields after surgery were normal. At presentation visual acuity was finger counting in the right eye and 20/20 in the left eye. There was marked loss of visual field in the right eye and a normal field in the left eye. Funduscopic appearance was normal.

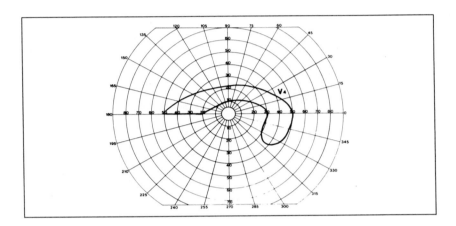

CT and magnetic resonance imaging scans showed no evidence of recurrence of the pituitary tumor, and the optic nerves appeared normal. Radiation vasculitis was presumed to be the cause of the optic neuropathy. The patient received hyperbaric oxygen therapy, but 2 months later vision in the left eye deteriorated to hand motion. The hyperbaric oxygen treatment was repeated, but no vision was restored.

This case represents the rare circumstance of optic nerve vasculitis following radiation therapy. The usual time course for the occurrence is 6 months to 2 years after the radiation. The precise mechanism is unknown. It is seen after routine, uncomplicated radiotherapy employing standard doses. A host susceptibility is postulated. Both eyes are frequently affected, and visual loss is usually severe. Corticosteroids have not been effective in treatment, but hyperbaric oxygen has been employed with some success.

Radiation optic neuropathy can also follow radiotherapy given for sinus and orbital lesions. In these cases swelling of the optic disk is usually noted, with marked leakage from the disk producing considerable retinal and subretinal exudation, as shown in Plate 28.

Bibliography

PAPILLOPHLEBITIS

Appen, R. E., de Venecia, G., and Ferwerda, J. Optic disk vasculitis. *Am. J. Ophthalmol.* 90:352, 1980.

Ellenberger, C., and Messner, K. H. Papillophlebitis: Benign retinopathy resembling papilledema or papillitis. *Ann. Neurol.* 3:438, 1978.

Miller, N. R. The Big Blind Spot Syndrome: Unilateral Optic Disc Edema Without Visual Loss or Increased Intracranial Pressure. In J. L. Smith (ed.), *Neuro-ophthalmology Update.* New York: Masson, 1977. Pp. 163–169.

PARTIAL CENTRAL RETINAL VEIN OCCLUSION

Hayreh, S. S. Central retinal vein occlusion: Differential diagnosis and management. *Trans. Am. Acad. Ophthalmol. Otolaryngol.* 83:379, 1977.

Zegarra, H., et al. Partial occlusion of the central retinal vein. *Am. J. Ophthalmol.* 96:330, 1983.

DIABETIC PAPILLOPATHY

Appen, R. E., et al. Diabetic papillopathy. *Am. J. Ophthalmol.* 90:203, 1980.

Barr, C. C., Glaser, J. S., Blankenship, G. Acute disc swelling in juvenile diabetes: Clinical profile and natural history of 12 cases. *Arch. Ophthalmol.* 98:2185, 1980.

Hayreh, S. S., and Zahoruk, R. M. Anterior ischemic optic neuropathy: VI. In juvenile diabetes. *Ophthalmologica* 182:13, 1981.

Lubow, M., and Makley, T. A. Pseudopapilledema of juvenile diabetes mellitus. *Arch. Ophthalmol.* 85:417, 1971.

Pavan, P. R., et al. Optic disc edema in juvenile-onset diabetes. *Arch. Ophthalmol.* 98:2193, 1980.

THYROID OPTIC NEUROPATHY

Feldon, S. E., et al. Quantitative computed tomography of Graves' ophthalmopathy: Extraocular muscle and orbital fat in development of optic neuropathy. *Arch. Ophthalmol.* 103:213, 1985.

Feldon, S. E., Muramatsu, S., Weiner, J. M. Clinical classification of Graves' ophthalmopathy: Identification of risk factors for optic neuropathy. *Arch. Ophthalmol.* 102:1469, 1984.

Kennerdell, J. S., Rosenbaum, A. E., and El-Hoshy, M. H. Apical optic nerve compression of dysthyroid optic neuropathy on computed tomography. *Arch. Ophthalmol.* 99:807, 1981.

Panzo, G. J., and Tomsak, R. L. A retrospective review of 26 cases of dysthyroid optic neuropathy. *Am. J. Ophthalmol.* 96:190, 1983.

Trobe, J. D., Glaser, J. S., and Laflamme, P. Dysthyroid optic neuropathy: Clinical profile and rationale for management. *Arch. Ophthalmol.* 96:1199, 1978.

SARCOID OPTIC NEUROPATHY

Beardsley, T. L., et al. Eleven cases of sarcoidosis of the optic nerve. *Am. J. Ophthalmol.* 97:62, 1984.

Caplan, L., et al. Neuro-ophthalmologic signs in the angiitic form of neuro-sarcoidosis. *Neurology* 33:1130, 1983.

Gudeman, S. K., et al. Sarcoid optic neuropathy. *Neurology.* 32:597, 1982.

OPTIC DISK INFARCT—6:45 SYNDROME

Lichter, P. R., and Henderson, J. W. Optic nerve infarction. *Am. J. Ophthalmol.* 85:302, 1978.

SHOCK OPTIC NEUROPATHY

Drance, S. M. The visual field of low tension glaucoma and shock-induced optic neuropathy. *Arch. Ophthalmol.* 95 : 1359, 1977.

Klewin, K. M., Appen, R. E., and Kaufman, P. L. Amaurosis and blood loss. *Am. J. Ophthalmol.* 86 : 669, 1978.

SYPHILIS

Rush, J. A., and Ryan, E. J. Syphilitic optic perineuritis. *Am. J. Ophthalmol.* 91 : 404, 1981.

Walsh, F. B. Syphilis of the optic nerve. *Trans. Am. Acad. Ophthalmol. Otolaryngol.* 60 : 39, 1956.

Weinstein, J. M., et al. Acute syphilitic optic neuritis. *Arch. Ophthalmol.* 99 : 1392, 1981.

RADIATION OPTIC NEUROPATHY

Brown, G. C., et al. Radiation optic neuropathy. *Ophthalmology* 89 : 1489, 1982.

Guy, J., and Schatz, N. J. Hyperbaric oxygen in the treatment of radiation-induced optic neuropathy. *Ophthalmology* 93 : 1083, 1986.

Harris, J. R., and Levene, M. B. Visual complications following irradiation for pituitary adenomas and craniopharyngiomas. *Radiology* 120 : 167, 1976.

17

Chiasmal Syndrome— Pituitary Tumor

A 32-year-old man was referred for neuro-ophthalmic evaluation after a screening optometric examination picked up bitemporal visual field loss. He had been examined 6 months earlier for unexplained anemia, and his medical history included loss of libido and generalized fatigue. He denied any symptoms of visual loss, diplopia, or headaches.

Neuro-Ophthalmic Examination

	OD	OS
Visual acuity	20/20	20/20
Color plates correct	12 of 12	12 of 12
Pupils	Normal	Normal
Lids, orbits, motility	Normal	Normal
Fundi	Normal	Normal

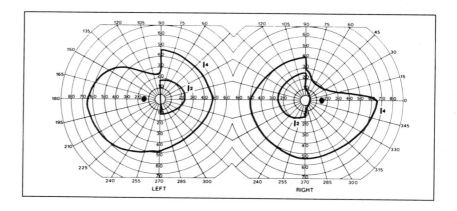

Summary
A 32-year-old man with a history of unexplained anemia and decreased libido was found on a routine eye exam to have bitemporal visual field defects.

Differential Diagnosis

Bitemporal visual field defects respecting the vertical meridian localize the disease to the optic chiasm. Occasionally, other disorders—congenitally tilted optic disks, papilledema with enlarged blind spots, nasal sector retinal lesions—may mimic a chiasmal syndrome by producing bitemporal visual field defects (see Fig. 1-13). However, the field defects in these disorders do not respect the vertical midline, and thus differentiation from a chiasmal syndrome should pose no diagnostic difficulty.

The most common cause of a chiasmal syndrome in an adult is a pituitary tumor. Craniopharyngioma, glioma, teratoma, aneurysm, mucocele, demyelinating disease, lymphoma, sarcoidosis, and metastases are less common causes. Although pituitary adenoma most often leads to symptomatic endocrine dysfunction, any of these lesions may lead to pituitary dysfunction through disruption of the hypothalamic-pituitary axis. Females who often present with amenorrhea or galactorrhea are more apt to manifest endocrine dysfunction than are males.

In this patient, the visual field defects unequivocally localized the disease to the optic chiasm. In addition he had symptoms suggestive of pituitary dysfunction. A pituitary tumor thus would be the most likely diagnosis.

Clinical Diagnosis: Chiasmal Syndrome, Probable Pituitary Tumor

Chiasmal compression can lead to a variety of visual field defects, as described in Chapter 1. Visual acuity may be normal or reduced. When the visual field loss in the two eyes is similar, the pupillary reactions will appear normal. However, with asymmetric involvement a relative afferent pupillary defect may be noted. With long-standing chiasmal compression, optic disk pallor may develop.

Patients may become aware of the visual field deficit but more often complain of a vague disturbance in visual function. Since opposite sides of the visual field are affected in each eye, binocularly the visual field remains fairly full until loss is extensive. With a complete bitemporal field defect, patients may note diplopia, which occurs from breakdown of an underlying phoria owing to a loss of fusion.

Pituitary tumors can be classified as secreting and nonsecreting. The nonsecreting tumors more often attain a large size and present with visual loss than do the secreting tumors, which tend to produce endocrine symptoms early and present when the tumor is still small. The exception is the prolactinoma in the male, in which chiasmal involvement is common at the time of presentation. In addition to prolactin, pituitary tumors may secrete growth hormone or corticotropin.

Less common manifestations of pituitary tumors include hydrocephalus and cavernous sinus involvement. The former occurs very rarely when the tumor enlarges to compress the third ventricle. The latter results when a pituitary tumor extends laterally into the cavernous sinus.

Cavernous sinus involvement may occur with or without chiasmal involvement. When lateral extension occurs, involvement of any or all of the nerves in the cavernous sinus (third, fourth, fifth [first division], sixth or sympathetics) is possible.

Additional Testing

In all cases, computed tomography (CT) or magnetic resonance imaging (MRI) scans of the area of the chiasm are necessary. On CT, coronal cuts may show a lesion better than routine axial cuts. Scans that are reported to be normal in cases of chiasmal syndromes generally have not been performed properly. The radiologist must be directed to examine the area of the chiasm rather than performing a routine scan through the entire brain. Even with proper scanning technique, occasionally the CT scan will appear normal. In these cases an MRI or metrizamide CT scan should be performed to obtain a better image of the chiasm. When a mass lesion is identified, a cerebral arteriogram or digital angiogram is generally indicated before surgery.

Treatment

Treatment of pituitary tumors is generally surgical. Medical therapy (bromocriptine mesylate) and radiation therapy may be considered as primary modalities in selected cases. Bromocriptine mesylate has been demonstrated to reduce the size of prolactin-secreting tumors. It has been less effective with other types of pituitary tumors. Bromocriptine mesylate has been employed as initial therapy in prolactinomas but may also be considered in the treatment of prolactinomas in which surgical resection has been subtotal. Radiation therapy as a primary modality should be considered only when surgery is contraindicated because of the patient's medical status.

The surgical approach to a pituitary tumor depends on the size of the tumor and the degree of upward extension. With tumors contained inferior to the optic chiasm, a transphenoidal approach is the procedure of choice. With extension into the suprasellar cistern and above, a subfrontal approach is generally necessary to visualize the chiasm directly in order to decompress it. With large tumors, a complete resection is generally not possible.

When there is residual tumor after surgery, radiation is generally administered.

Management and Course of the Case

A CT scan demonstrated a 2-cm mass extending superiorly from the region of the sella into the suprasellar cistern with obliteration of the chiasmal contour.

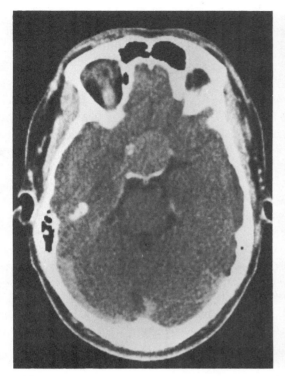

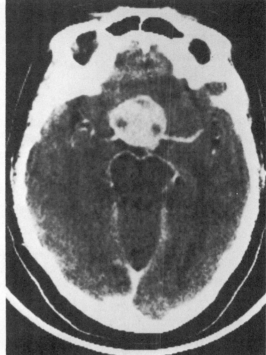

Without contrast   *With contrast*

Endocrine studies revealed a prolactin level of 4000 mU per ml and a slightly depressed serum testosterone level. Serum cortisol and growth hormone levels were normal as were results of thyroid function studies. The patient underwent a frontal craniotomy with a gross total resection of the tumor. After recovery from surgery, radiation therapy was carried out. By 10 weeks after surgery, the patient's prolactin level had decreased to 65 mU per ml and his visual field deficits had cleared entirely. With monthly testosterone shots and low-dose bromocriptine mesylate the patient has been asymptomatic for the 2 years since surgery.

Pituitary Apoplexy

A 62-year-old man noted the abrupt onset of headache and blurred vision. Six months earlier he had been seen for a right temporal field defect and was diagnosed as having ischemic optic neuropathy. His medical history was unremarkable. Visual acuity was 20/30 in the right eye and 20/20 in the left eye, with a right relative afferent pupillary defect. Funduscopy showed nerve fiber layer loss in the retina in both eyes, but the optic disks appeared normal.

As can be seen, the visual fields clearly indicated chiasmal involvement. The previous diagnosis of ischemic optic neuropathy had been made erroneously. On CT, there was evidence of a large suprasellar mass consistent with pituitary tumor. Cerebral angiography demonstrated that the mass extended superiorly from the region of the sella with encasement of the internal carotid arteries on the right greater than on the left.

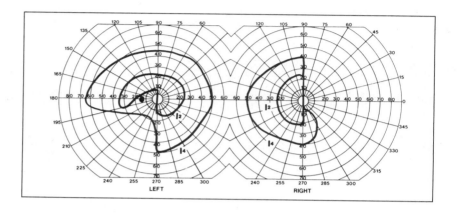

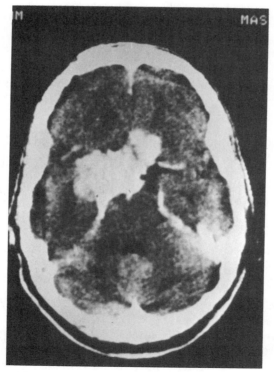

With contrast

A diagnosis of pituitary apoplexy was made. The patient was given hydrocortisone replacement urgently. His endocrine function tests demonstrated panhypopituitarism. At surgery a large hemorrhagic necrotic pituitary adenoma was grossly removed with postoperative radiation treatment. Receiving thyroid, cortisone, and testosterone replacement therapy, he is asymptomatic with residual unchanged visual field defects 2 years after surgery.

First described in 1950 by Brougham and colleagues, the concept of pituitary apoplexy has become well defined. This syndrome represents hemorrhage into a pituitary tumor, which is usually of moderate or large size at the time of the bleed. The manifestations of pituitary apoplexy depend on the direction of expansion of the swollen necrotic pituitary gland. A sudden severe headache is a typical presenting symptom. Symptoms may evolve over a period of 24 to 48 hours, although we have seen progression over a period of weeks. Compression of the chiasm, one or both cavernous sinuses, or all of these occurs in the typical case, producing rapid visual loss, ophthalmoplegia, or both. In addition there may be impaired consciousness or vegetative signs from involvement of the diencephalon and midbrain. With enough lateral expansion, there may be compression of the carotid arteries with secondary cortical infarction. Rarely, there will be expansion inferiorly with resultant epistaxis. Signs of meningitis may also develop as the necrotic tissue exudes into the subarachnoid space.

The initial treatment of pituitary apoplexy consists of hormonal replacement, followed by surgical resection of the tumor. High-dose corticosteroids should be administered as soon as the diagnosis is made. When visual loss has occurred, decompression of the tumor should be performed as soon as the patient's medical condition is stabilized.

Chiasmal Demyelination

A 24-year-old dance student developed visual blurring and a numb right leg over a 7-day period while on tour in Europe. Neuro-ophthalmic examination revealed visual acuity of 20/40 in each eye. Color vision was normal with Ishihara plates. Both pupils were sluggishly reactive. Funduscopic findings were normal. On general neurologic examination there was incoordination of the right leg and bilateral Babinski responses. Her visual field is shown below. Routine CT scan was normal, but because a compressive lesion of the chiasm was suspected, a metrizamide CT scan of the suprasellar region was performed. It also was normal. Magnetic resonance imaging demonstrated multiple periventricular regions of water density which suggested the diagnosis of a demyelinating process (see p. 128). Cerebrospinal fluid showed a slightly elevated protein of 48 mg/100 ml with positive oligoclonal banding and an elevated level of myelin basic protein.

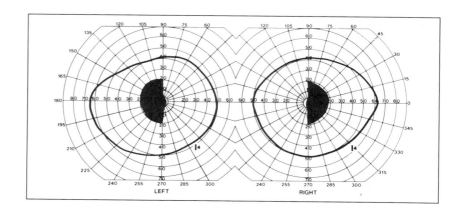

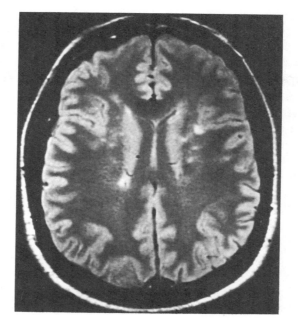

The patient was not treated. One month after her initial presentation her visual field had returned to normal.

Demyelinating disease rarely presents as a chiasmal syndrome. The diagnosis of multiple sclerosis in a patient with a bitemporal field defect mandates excluding all other causes of chiasmal compression or infiltration.

Bitemporal Defects from Tilted Optic Disks

A 29-year-old man noted occasional trouble seeing when looking over his shoulder to back his car out of the garage. He denied headaches, and although he had always had "thick glasses," he had never had problems seeing with his glasses. Visual acuity was 20/20 in each eye with a myopic correction.

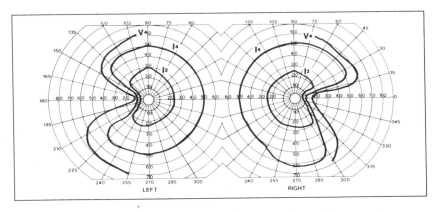

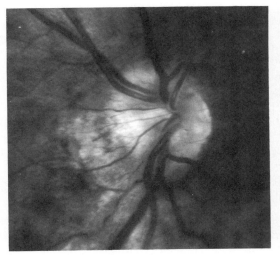
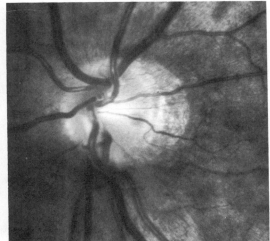

OD   OS

The visual field defects can be seen to extend to the blind spot and not to the vertical midline. Because of this, a chiasmal lesion should not be a consideration. The optic disk appearance indicates congenital tilted optic disks.

Of course, patients with tilted optic disks are not protected from developing central nervous system (CNS) tumors, and if a patient has symptoms suggesting a CNS lesion, the appropriate neuroimaging should be done even if the visual field fits the funduscopic picture.

A 60-year-old man noted visual blurring while working at his word processor. His health had been excellent; he had not undergone an eye examination in over 20 years.

Visual acuity was 20/20 in each eye. Visual field defects were present, as can be seen below. Intraocular pressure was 35 mm Hg in each eye. Funduscopy showed marked cupping of both optic disks.

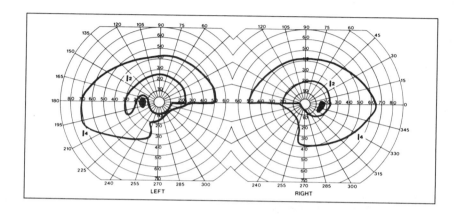

The visual field shows marked loss of the nasal field in both eyes. This pattern is almost never due to an intracranial lesion; rather optic disk disease is usually present. Lateral compression of the chiasm on both sides producing binasal defects is exceedingly rare. Binasal field loss can be seen in functional field deficits, but this is rare. Glaucoma was the diagnosis in this case.

Bibliography

Adler, F. H., Austin, G., and Grant, F. C. Localizing value of visual fields in patients with early chiasmal lesions. *Arch. Ophthalmol.* 40:579, 1948.

Bird, A. C. Field loss due to lesions at the anterior angle of the chiasm. *Proc. R. Soc. Med.* 65:519, 1972.

David, N. J., Gargano, F. P., and Glaser, J. S. Pituitary Apoplexy in Clinical Perspective. In J. S. Glaser and J. L. Smith (eds.), *Neuro-Ophthalmology*, Vol. 8. St. Louis: Mosby, 1975. Pp. 140–165.

Hollenhorst, R. W., and Younge, B. R. Ocular Manifestations Produced by Adenomas of the Pituitary Gland: Analysis of 1,000 Cases. In P. O. Kohler and G. T. Ross (eds.), *Diagnosis and Treatment of Pituitary Tumors*. New York: Elsevier, 1973. Pp. 53–64.

Hoyt, W. F. Correlative functional anatomy of the optic chiasm—1969. *Clin. Neurosurg.* 17:189, 1970.

Kennedy, H. B., and Smith, R. J. S. Eye signs in craniopharyngioma. *Br. J. Ophthalmol.* 59:689, 1975.

Moster, M. L., et al. Visual function in prolactinoma patients treated with brom-ocriptine. *Ophthalmology* 92:1332, 1985.

Newman, S. A. Advances in diagnosis and treatment of pituitary tumors. *Int. Ophthalmol. Clin.* 26 (4): 285, 1986.

Reid, R. L., Quigly, M. E., and Yen, S. S. C. Pituitary apoplexy: A review. *Arch. Neurol.* 42:712, 1985.

Rovit, R. L., and Fein, J. M. Pituitary apoplexy: A review and reappraisal. *J. Neurosurg.* 37:280, 1972.

Sacks, J. G., and Melen, O. Bitemporal visual field defects in presumed multiple sclerosis. *J.A.M.A.* 234:69, 1975.

Spector, R. H., Glaser, J. S., and Schatz, N. J. Demyelinating chiasmal lesions. *Arch. Neurol.* 37:757, 1980.

Unsold, R., and Hoyt, W. F. Band atrophy of the optic nerve. *Arch. Ophthalmol.* 98:1637, 1980.

Wakai, S., et al. Pituitary apoplexy: Its incidence and clinical significance. *J. Neurosurg.* 55:187, 1981.

Weinberger, L. M., Adler, F. H., and Grant, F. C. Primary pituitary adenoma and the syndrome of the cavernous sinus: A clinical and anatomic study. *Arch. Ophthalmol.* 24:1197, 1940.

18

Optic Tract Syndrome

A 56-year-old fisherman presented with a complaint of "glare" in his left visual field. The previous summer he had noted difficulty navigating his fishing boat through a rocky channel. He denied headaches, diplopia, change in hair growth, or loss of libido. Results of a general neurologic examination and routine computed tomography (CT) scan of the head had been reported as normal 8 months previously.

Neuro-Ophthalmic Examination

	OD	OS
Visual acuity	20/20	20/40
Color plates correct	12 of 12	8 of 12
Pupils	Normal	Relative afferent pupillary defect
Lids, orbits, motility	Normal	Normal
Fundi	Normal	Normal

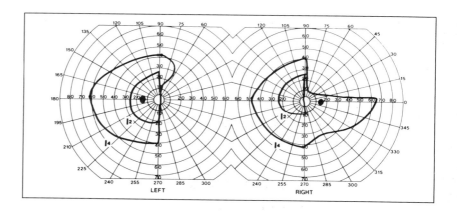

A general neurologic examination was normal.

Summary

A 56-year-old man with a complaint of mildly obscured vision was found to have an incongruous homonymous hemianopia.

Differential Diagnosis

The incongruous homonymous hemianopia, reduced central visual acuity, and relative afferent pupillary defect in this patient localize the lesion to the optic tract. The optic tract is formed by visual fibers that extend from the posterior portion of the optic chiasm to synapse in the lateral geniculate nucleus. The tracts diverge from the chiasm to sweep around the cerebral peduncles, deriving their vascular supply from penetrating branches of the middle cerebral artery. Because the optic tract is rarely involved without contiguous involvement of the optic nerve, chiasm, or cerebral peduncles, it is more appropriate to speak of an optic tract syndrome than an optic tract lesion.

The optic tract syndrome is characterized, as in this patient, by an incongruous homonymous hemianopia, relative afferent pupillary defect, and the variable presence of optic atrophy. When optic atrophy has had time to develop, it will take on the pattern of homonymous hemioptic atrophy. A relative afferent pupillary defect is detected in approximately 80 percent of cases of optic tract involvement. The defect is usually present in the eye on the same side as the lesion but occasionally is present on the opposite side, depending on which eye has the greater amount of visual field loss.

The more frequently encountered pathologic entities leading to this syndrome are craniopharyngioma, pituitary tumor, aneurysm, and demyelinating disease.

In this patient the presence of an optic tract syndrome with a lack of endocrine or other contiguous neurologic signs favors the diagnosis of craniopharyngioma.

Clinical Diagnosis: Optic Tract Syndrome, Probable Craniopharyngioma

As with chiasmal compression, the patient with an optic tract syndrome often complains of a vague disturbance in visual function. This may be described as glare, as seen with this patient, or a "washout" of colors and fine detail—symptoms often difficult for the clinician to pinpoint, a factor resulting in delays in establishing a diagnosis.

Craniopharyngiomas arise from nests of squamous epithelial cells that are the remnants of Rathke's pouch lying between the anterior and posterior lobes of the pituitary gland. Although they may develop at any age, craniopharyngiomas are most commonly found in children. When craniopharyngiomas are present in adults, the clinical manifestations are progressive field loss often associated with endocrine disturbances and dementia. Although a bitemporal hemianopia is the most common visual field deficit seen in craniopharyngioma, incongruous homonymous hemianopia of optic tract origin is frequently seen.

Additional Testing

Neuroimaging studies in craniopharyngioma may demonstrate calcium within the tumor; however, as with this patient, the large cystic component may elude CT detection. Thus either magnetic resonance imaging (MRI) studies or a metrizamide CT scan of the suprasellar cistern may be needed.

Treatment

The treatment of craniopharyngioma is controversial. Our approach is decompression of the optic tract or chiasm from the surgical approach that best permits visualization of the tumor mass, followed by a course of radiation therapy. Despite this type of combined therapy, recurrence is the rule, and the patient should be followed with serial perimetry and MRI.

Management and Course of the Case

On repeat CT scanning, suprasellar calcium was noted with distortion of the normal chiasmal contour. Metrizamide CT scan confirmed the presence of a suprasellar cystic lesion. Endocrine studies had normal results. At surgery a craniopharyngioma was found and partly resected. Postoperatively, a course of radiation was carried out. After the radiation therapy the patient's vision was 20/20 in each eye with full visual fields and normal color vision. Six months postoperatively his vision dropped in the left eye, and repeat CT scanning demonstrated recurrence of the cystic component. He was referred for radioactive seed implantation.

Optic Tract Demyelination

A 34-year-old man was found confused with a bitten tongue and periods of incontinence. On arrival in the emergency room he was coherent but complaining of a headache. He gave a history of a similar episode of loss of consciousness 2 years previously. At that time he had been found to have a normal electroencephalogram and a CT scan that showed a "low density region" in the right cortex that resolved on subsequent scanning. He also reported having had transient unexplained diplopia and urinary urgency 4 years previously. Visual acuity was 20/30 on the right and 20/20 on the left with a right relative afferent pupillary defect. Funduscopy showed nerve fiber layer loss in the retina in both eyes but normal-appearing optic disks. Ocular motility and the results of a general neurologic examination were normal.

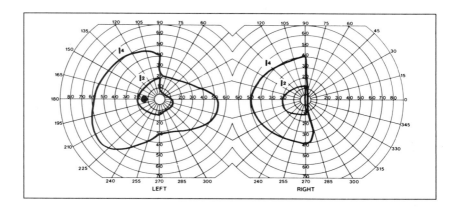

These visual fields, when coupled with the patient's decreased visual acuity and relative afferent pupillary defect on the right, indicate a left optic tract syndrome. The additional history of diplopia and urinary symptoms suggests the presence of previous insults to the white matter of the central nervous system consistent with a diagnosis of multiple sclerosis (MS). MRI confirmed the presence of multiple water-density lesions consistent with the diagnosis of MS.

The patient was treated with phenytoin (Dilantin) for control of seizures. Over the course of 4 weeks the visual field defect cleared entirely, as did the relative afferent pupillary defect. One year later he returned with a left hemiparesis and internuclear ophthalmoplegia.

The optic tract syndrome, as with the chiasmal syndrome, is rarely the sole presentation of a demyelinating process. Prudence mandates establishing the diagnosis of MS through MRI and cerebrospinal fluid analysis.

Bibliography

Bell, R. A., and Thompson, H. S. Relative afferent pupillary defect in optic tract hemianopias. *Am. J. Ophthalmol.* 85:538, 1978.

Bender, M. B., and Bodis-Wollner, I. Visual dysfunction in optic tract lesions. *Ann. Neurol.* 3:187, 1978.

Newman, S. A., and Miller, N. R. Optic tract syndrome: Neuro-ophthalmic considerations. *Arch. Ophthalmol.* 101:1241, 1983.

O'Connor, P. S., et al. The Marcus Gunn pupil in experimental optic tract lesions. *Ophthalmology,* 89:160, 1982.

Savino, P. J., et al. Optic tract syndrome: A review of 21 patients. *Arch. Ophthalmol.* 96:656, 1978.

19

Homonymous Hemianopia

A 47-year-old woman was seen after the abrupt onset of a scintillating scotoma in the right visual field that lasted 20 minutes and was followed by a severe left retro-orbital headache. Her medical history was unremarkable: There was no history of hypertension, migraine headache, or diabetes.

Neuro-Ophthalmic Examination

	OD	OS
Visual acuity	20/20	20/20
Color plates correct	12 of 12	12 of 12
Pupils	Normal	Normal
Motility, lids, orbits	Normal	Normal
Fundi	Normal	Normal

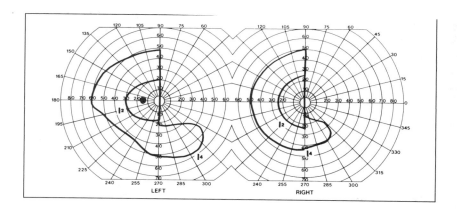

Symmetric optokinetic nystagmus (OKN) was present. Results of a neurologic exam were normal.

Summary

A 47-year-old woman had the abrupt onset of a congruous right homonymous hemianopia and no associated neurologic findings.

Differential Diagnosis

A homonymous hemianopia may occur with a lesion anywhere in the visual system from the optic tract through the occipital lobe. The diagnosis of optic tract involvement is detailed in Chapter 18. Localization in the retrogeniculate system can often be determined based on the pattern of the visual field defects and the OKN response.

Temporal lobe lesions tend to produce visual field defects affecting the superior field, while parietal lobe lesions produce defects that are either complete or more dense inferiorly. Occipital lobe lesions are characterized by field defects that are very congruous between the two eyes. The macular representation and temporal crescent may be either solely involved or spared.

The OKN response may help differentiate an occipital from a parietal lesion. Optokinetic nystagmus is typically symmetric into the two visual fields with lesions involving the occipital cortex; it is only with lesions of the deep parietal region that the optokinetic fiber pathways are disrupted, leading to a deficit of the ipsilateral slow component.

In this patient, the complete congruity of the visual field defect, coupled with the otherwise normal neurologic findings and symmetry of the OKN response, suggests the presence of an occipital lobe lesion. The abruptness of onset and presence of headache further suggest a vascular lesion with the possibility of an intraparenchymal hemorrhage into the occipital lobe.

The presence of positive visual phenomena (scintillating scotoma in this case) indicates afferent visual system irritation, which may occur from the retina to the occipital cortex. Vitreoretinal traction typically produces small flashes that flicker for seconds at a time. Large scintillations that last several minutes or longer generally indicate an occipital origin. Although most typical of migraine, a scintillating scotoma may occur with other occipital processes such as hemorrhage, arteriovenous malformation, tumor, or infarction.

Clinical Diagnosis: Occipital Lobe Lesion

Lesions involving the occipital cortex can be diagnosed based on pathognomonic visual field findings:

1. Congruity of the homonymous defects
2. Temporal crescent preservation
3. Macular sparing
4. Cortical blindness

Congruity of a visual field defect implies a lesion placed posteriorly in the optic radiations. The fibers of the optic radiations become completely segregated when the visual cortex is reached; the signature of an occipital lesion is precise congruity of the homonymous defects. This is true whether the field defect is quadrantic or a homonymous scotoma.

In the complete homonymous hemianopias congruity cannot be ascertained, and thus the lesion cannot be localized.

The visual cortex lying anteriorly in the interhemispheric fissure corresponds to the peripheralmost nasal retina representation. With infarction of the occipital cortex this anterior portion may be spared (through collateral arterial supply from the anterior circulation), leading to residual vision in the extreme of the temporal field contralaterally. Similarly, the temporal crescent region may be selectively damaged, leading to a monocular temporal visual field deficit. This is quite rare.

Macular sparing may be due to either a dual arterial supply to the occipital pole from middle and posterior cerebral artery branches or bilateral retinal ganglion cell projection to the macular region.

Cortical blindness results from the destruction of both occipital lobes, usually from bilateral infarctions caused by vertebral basilar disease or as a complication of hypotension. Cortical blindness is characterized by blindness in the setting of normal pupillary reflexes and absent OKN response. Whatever visual field remains will be identical in the two eyes.

The more common lesions of the occipital lobe are vascular from either thrombotic infarction or intraparenchymal hemorrhage. Infarction in this region is from branch posterior cerebral artery thrombosis, an embolus from the vertebral basilar system, vasospasm from migraine, or vasculitis. Hemorrhages can be a result of thrombosis, embolism, or arteriovenous malformations that may or may not show up on neuroimaging studies.

Additional Testing

Computed tomography (CT) scanning will delineate the nature of the damage in occipital lobe disease, and arteriography may be indicated to look for an underlying source of embolism or vascular malformation. With ischemic infarction of the occipital lobe, the CT scan may be normal immediately but typically demonstrates a region of low density within 48 to 72 hours. Using intravenous contrast enhancement with CT scanning increases the yield of early detection of the infarct through the enhancement of regions of blood-brain barrier breakdown. Magnetic resonance imaging may be a more sensitive test for detecting early infarction without the morbidity associated with the injection of contrast material. Electroencephalography has little place in the anatomic localization of occipital cortex disease, with the rare exception of the patient with formed repetitive visual hallucinations who is suspected of having focal seizures.

Treatment

The management of occipital lobe infarction or hemorrhage depends on the age of the patient, presence of associated neurologic findings, and the cause of the vascular event. In the case of a hemorrhage, we admit the patient for close observation to treat any swelling around the region of hemorrhage. In the case of an otherwise asymptomatic occipital lobe infarct, the evaluation should consist of blood pressure measurement (both arms—to rule out subclavian steal syndrome); blood glucose, cholesterol, and triglyceride determinations; and a thorough cardiac evaluation for the presence of an embolic source and other associated atherosclerotic disease. Consideration for arteriography should be made on an individual basis. When the cause is clearly posterior circulation small vessel disease in an elderly patient with known atherosclerosis elsewhere, little else needs to be done beyond starting antiplatelet therapy and counseling the patient not to drive.

The prognosis for occipital lobe visual field defects depends on the underlying vascular pathophysiology. Generally, visual field loss from intraparenchymal hematomas clears more completely than the loss from infarction, because the majority of the dysfunction is from reversible swelling in the former, as opposed to the irreversible changes occurring with the latter.

Management and Course of the Case
CT scan demonstrated a blood-density lesion involving the left occipital region with extension into the parietal lobe. Arteriography demonstrated mass effect only. The right homonymous hemianopia gradually resolved with a residual small right homonymous scotoma. One year after the initial hemorrhage the patient had another hemorrhage involving the same region, with recurrence of the right homonymous hemianopia and concurrent mild dysphasia. A repeat arteriogram was unremarkable. Eighteen months after the initial event she experienced a third left parietal-occipital hemorrhage, which produced dense aphasia and right homonymous hemianopia.

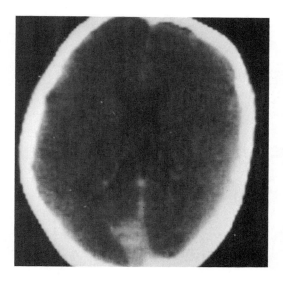

Recurrent intraparenchymal brain hemorrhage in the setting of a normal blood pressure and no arteriographic evidence of vascular malformation should suggest the diagnosis of cerebral amyloid angiopathy. There is no treatment for this condition, other than supportive, and it has an unknown natural history.

Cortical Blindness

A 69-year-old man noted the abrupt onset of decreased vision in his right hemifield. On examination he was found to have a right homonymous visual field defect. Three months later his vision abruptly became more blurred while watching television. He denied headache and had no other neurologic symptoms. He had a history of long-standing hypertension and diabetes mellitus. Visual acuity was 20/50 in each eye with a small area of right macular field and an area of left superior field spared. In addition there was sparing of the left temporal crescent. CT scanning demonstrated bilateral occipital lobe infarcts.

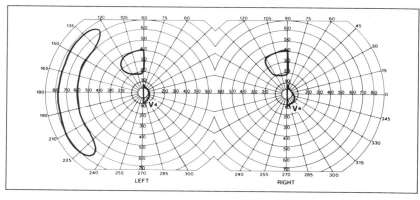

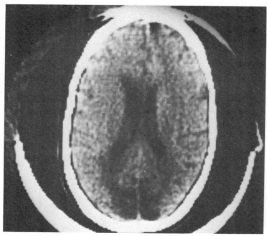

Although this case might be mistaken for optic nerve or retinal disease producing decreased acuity and the field defects outlined, it is a classic example of bilateral occipital lobe disease with asymmetric paired bilateral incomplete hemianopias. In optic nerve or retinal disease the monocular field defects do not respect the vertical meridian, whereas in bilateral occipital lobe disease the defects form a step across the vertical and are identical in the two eyes.

Homonymous Hemianopia from Parietal Lobe Lesion

A 58-year-old man noted blurred vision to the left. He had experienced progressive right-sided headaches over the preceding 4 months. His medical history was otherwise unremarkable.

On examination he had a fairly congruous left inferior quadrantanopsia. The OKN response was decreased with the tape moving to the right. On neurologic examination he demonstrated left body and visual space neglect (which made perimetry quite difficult).

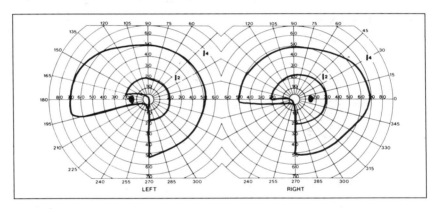

This patient presents a classic picture of right parietal lobe dysfunction with an inferior quadrantic field defect and left body space neglect on examination. The CT scan confirmed the presence of a right parietal enhancing lesion, which was found to be a high-grade glioma at the time of surgery.

Nondominant parietal lobe lesions typically present only after a considerable degree of damage has occurred to that area of the cortex. When these patients do come in for evaluation, their prominent body space neglect and unusual affect obscure the extent of visual field dysfunction. Optokinetic nystagmus may be diminished into the field of vision ipsilateral to the cortical lesion because of interruption of the pathways subserving this modality.

Dominant parietal lobe lesions are more easily picked up clinically with their concomitant language dysfunction or Gerstmann's syndrome (finger agnosia, right-left confusion, agraphia, acalculia) as well as the right inferior or complete homonymous hemianopia.

Visual field testing in parietal lobe lesions is frequently frustrating because patient fixation is often difficult to maintain. Parietal lobe lesions are more often the result of an infarct than a tumor as was found in this case.

Homonymous Hemianopia from Temporal Lobe Lesion

A 22-year-old female college volleyball star had episodes of déjà vu that came on with exercise. She had noted difficulty in hitting her shots to the right side over the past year.

Visual acuity was 20/20 in both eyes with good pupillary reflexes and normal fundi. Results of a general neurologic exam and an awake-sleep electroencephalogram were normal. Results of Goldmann perimetry are shown below.

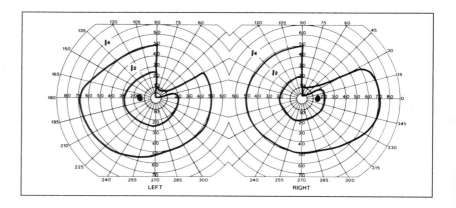

This patient's symptoms and perimetry findings suggest left temporal lobe disease. A CT scan demonstrated an enhancing midtemporal lobe mass on the left. Arteriography showed no evidence of a vascular malformation or mass effect.

Because of increasing focal seizures refractory to conventional anticonvulsant therapy, she underwent a left craniotomy with resection of the mass using concomitant language mapping intraoperatively. Histologically, the tumor was found to be a low-grade astrocytoma. Her examination results remained unchanged postoperatively, and she is now seizure free.

After leaving the lateral geniculate nucleus the visual fibers subserving the superior visual field course anteriorly around the temporal horn, forming Meyer's loop. These fibers run in close proximity to the internal capsule and temporal isthmus. The hallmark of the temporal lobe lesion is the homonymous superior quadrantopsia with or without the associated neurologic findings of aphasia, motor or sensory deficits, or seizures. Although there is debate in the literature about the congruity of these field defects, in our experience when perimetry is performed by a careful perimetrist, the defects are often more dense in the eye on the side of the lesion.

Bibliography

Aldrich, M. S., et al. Cortical blindness: Etiology, diagnosis, and prognosis. *Ann. Neurol.* 21:149, 1987.

Anderson, D. R. *Testing the Field of Vision.* St. Louis: Mosby, 1982.

Ask-Upmark, E. On the cortical projection of the temporal half-moon of the visual field. *Acta Ophthalmol. (Copenh.)* 10:271, 1932.

Benton, S., Levy, I., and Swash, M. Vision in the temporal crescent in occipital infarction. *Brain* 103:83, 1980.

Bunt, A. H., and Minckler, D. S. Foveal sparing. *Arch. Ophthalmol.* 95:1445, 1977.

Holmes, G. Disturbances of vision by cerebral lesions. *Br. J. Ophthalmol.* 2:353, 1918.

Parkinson, D., and Craig, W. Tumours of the brain, occipital lobe: Their signs and symptoms. *Can. Med. Assoc. J.* 64:111, 1951.

Spector, R. H., et al. Occipital lobe infarctions: Perimetry and computed tomography. *Neurology* 31:1098, 1981.

Traquair, H. M. *An Introduction to Clinical Perimetry* (3rd ed.). St. Louis: Mosby, 1940.

Trobe, J. D., and Glaser, J. S. *The Visual Field Manual.* Gainesville, Fla.: Triad, 1983.

Walsh, T. J. Temporal crescent or half-moon syndrome. *Ann. Ophthalmol.* 6:501, 1974.

20

Migraine

A 21-year-old woman noted episodic visual blurring lasting 15 to 30 minutes. These episodes consisted of a bright "blurring light" in the central aspect of her visual field that gradually spread to the periphery, with a perception of multicolored zigzag lines shimmering "like sunlight reflecting off the surface of water." At the end of an episode she would develop a dimness in the involved hemifield associated with a variable speech and hemisensory disturbance. The entire episode would last approximately 1 hour. Episodes occurred several times per month but with an increased frequency just before the onset of menses. She denied any associated headaches but did note that she always had an upset stomach after the visual episodes.

Results of her neuro-ophthalmic examination were entirely normal.

Summary
A young woman with paroxysmal episodes of visual distortion associated with transient sensory and speech disturbances was found to have normal examination results.

Differential Diagnosis
The occurrence of stereotyped repetitive hemifield visual hallucinations associated with cortical symptoms of speech and sensory disturbance suggests a disturbance of cerebral cortex rather than retina. Paroxysmal events occurring at a cortical level are usually vasospastic, ischemic, or epileptic. Their occurrence in a young adult without other evidence of vascular disease, and no other stigmata of seizure disorder, suggests transient episodes of vasospasm. Other considerations include occipital lobe arteriovenous malformation (AVM), coagulopathy, and systemic vasculitis. Occipital tumors or AVM may cause migrainelike visual symptoms, but the pattern of visual distortion is usually more brief and fortification spectra are less well formed than in classic migraine (see Arteriovenous Malformation Mimicking Migraine, below).

A common problem seen in our clinics is the case of transient visual distortion without accompanying findings on clinical or neuroimaging examinations. In the younger patients these symptoms are usually considered to be due to a migraine equivalent.

Clinical Diagnosis: Acephalgic Migraine ("Migraine Equivalents")

The scintillating scotoma is one of the more common paroxysmal visual phenomena and is thought to occur through spreading cortical depression when ischemia occurs in the posterior circulation of the brain. This ischemia may be secondary to the transient vasospasm present with migraine, or it may be from primary vascular disease with atherosclerotic vascular changes, embolism, or vasculitis. When followed by a headache these symptoms are almost always diagnostic of migraine. However, even without headache, in a young individual migraine is the likely diagnosis. In this setting the symptom complex is referred to as acephalgic migraine or migraine equivalents.

Virtually any cortical region may be involved with focal ischemia secondary to vasospasm; the resultant bewildering array of transient focal neurologic signs and symptoms often leads the unwary clinician on unnecessary diagnostic witch-hunts. A careful history in these patients will usually uncover the stereotyped nature of the spells, past true migraine headaches, family history of migraine, and lack of fixed neurologic deficits despite repeated episodes.

Fisher has popularized the concept of transient migraine equivalents in middle-aged and older persons: transient neurologic signs or symptoms that occur in patients over the age of 40 not found to have obvious vascular disease and assumed to have vasospasm from migraine. In these patients there is a typical progression of migraine phenomena with or without the accompanying headache. We agree that many older patients presenting with scintillating scotoma with or without other focal neurologic symptoms or headache may have acephalgic migraine, but we would urge either close follow-up of these patients or, at the least, noninvasive neuroimaging studies to check the integrity of the vascular supply.

Additional Testing

The patient who presents with his or her first migraine equivalent will need careful consideration to rule out a treatable vascular basis for the symptoms before the event is labeled a migraine equivalent. If there is no history of headaches or family history of migraine (often present in individuals with migraine equivalents), we investigate as we would in a case of transient ischemic attack—with a vascular evaluation (blood pressure determination and cardiac ultrasound), as well as a contrast-enhanced computed tomography scan or magnetic resonance imaging scan of the head. Screening blood chemistry studies, complete blood count, serology, and antinuclear antibody screen should complete the evaluation to rule out systemic medical causes of vasculopathy. The decision regarding cerebral arteriography should be individualized.

Treatment

The treatment of migraine equivalents depends on the frequency of the episodes and can be aimed at either preventing the attacks or aborting them once in progress. When episodes occur with a frequency of less than once a month, we will often just start the patient on low-dose aspirin and follow him or her. If they occur more frequently, then we treat them as we do classic or common migraine with prophylactic medication, in addition to aspirin. In patients who have no medical contraindication to taking a beta blocker, we usually start with propranolol hydrochloride (20–40 mg) given two or three times daily, or a long-acting agent 80 mg once a day. This may be all that is needed to gain control of the episodes. In those patients who cannot tolerate propranolol hydrochloride we try a tricyclic antidepressant (amitriptyline), starting with a dose of 25 to 50 mg given just before sleep, and gradually increasing this to tolerance or abatement of the symptoms. Calcium channel blockers recently have been used with success.

Treatment to abort acephalgic migraine with ergotamine preparations, which promote vasoconstriction, is controversial and in our opinion not advisable.

Discontinuation of birth control pills should be considered in women who have migraine equivalents.

Management and Course of the Case

Further history obtained from the family revealed that the patient's mother and maternal grandmother had experienced similar episodes in their twenties. The patient desired no additional testing and was placed on a regimen of propranolol hydrochloride 40 mg twice daily with total abatement of her symptoms. Neuroimaging studies were not performed.

Arteriovenous Malformation Mimicking Migraine

A 32-year-old woman with a 5-year history of recurrent right lower quadrant visual field "light flashes" had a severe headache and persistent right visual field loss. Her visual symptoms typically lasted 20 to 30 minutes, were present in both eyes, and were accompanied by a variable headache. She had no family history of migraine, and conventional migraine therapy had not changed the frequency or severity of her symptoms. Her examination results were normal with the exception of the visual field defect shown on p. 147.

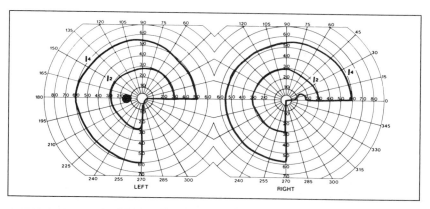

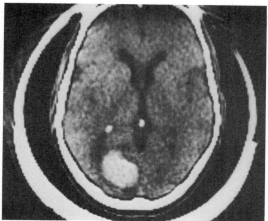

The visual field defect corresponds to the region of intraparenchymal hemorrhage. A cerebral angiogram confirmed the presence of an AVM. Although, as mentioned above, the visual symptoms seen in occipital lobe AVM are usually briefer and have less in the way of fortification spectra than in migraine, they may, as in this patient, be indistinguishable from those of classic migraine. The history of recurrent migraine-like events refractory to conventional therapy and occurring always on one side should have led to earlier neuroimaging in this patient.

Bibliography

Corbett, J. J. Neuro-ophthalmic complications of headaches. *Neurol. Clin.* 1: 973, 1983.

Fisher, C. M. Late-life migraine accompaniments as a cause of unexplained transient ischemic attacks. *Can. J. Neurol. Sci.* 7:9, 1980.

O'Connor, P. S., and Tredici, T. J. Acephalgic migraine: Fifteen years experience. *Ophthalmology* 88:999, 1981.

Troost, B. T., and Newton, T. H. Occipital lobe arteriovenous malformation: Clinical and radiologic features in 26 cases with comments on the differentiation from migraine. *Arch. Ophthalmol.* 93:250, 1975.

21

Functional Visual Loss

A 17-year-old girl complained of "tunnel vision," which had been present since an automobile accident in which she had killed a pedestrian.

Neuro-Ophthalmic Examination

	OD	OS
Visual acuity	20/20	20/20
Color plates correct	12 of 12	12 of 12
Pupils	Normal	Normal
Lids, orbits, motility	Normal	Normal
Fundi	Normal	Normal

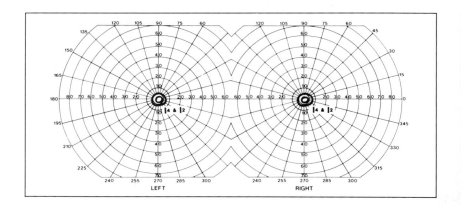

Summary

A 17-year-old girl had constricted visual fields and otherwise normal neuro-ophthalmic examination results.

Differential Diagnosis

The differential diagnosis of a grossly constricted visual field includes end-stage glaucoma, retinitis pigmentosa, chronic papilledema, bilateral homonymous hemianopia with macular sparing from bilateral occipital lobe disease, and functional constriction (hysterical or malingering).

With an organic cause of visual field constriction, the field will expand as the testing distance is increased. With functional constriction, this expansion does not occur, and thus the field at the various distances appears tubular (see below). In addition, on perimetry all isopters tend to fall close to (or cross) each other in the patient with functional constriction, whereas with organic disease there will be a separation between the isopters. Some patients with functional constriction will show spiraling on perimetry—that is, the field gradually expands as the perimetrist moves the target circumferentially.

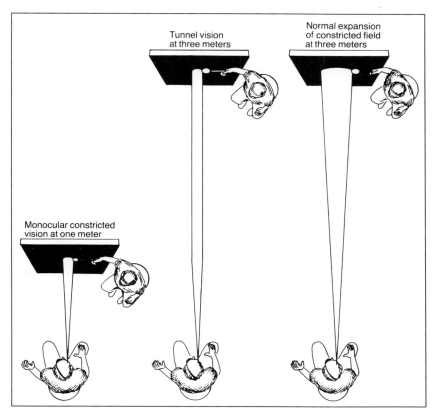

From C. H. Smith and R. W. Beck. Functional disease in neuro-ophthalmology. Neurol. Clin. 1 : 955, 1983. Reprinted with permission from W. B. Saunders Co.

Occipital lesions leading to constricted visual fields are readily identified by the irregular edge aligned along the vertical or horizontal meridian or both on perimetry. The remaining organic causes of constricted visual field can be readily identified by a careful funduscopic examination and by the physiologic expansion of the field at increasing distances.

In this patient the objective examination results were normal, and perimetry confirmed the presence of functional visual field constriction.

Clinical Diagnosis: Functional Visual Loss

Afferent or efferent visual system complaints are not infrequently found to be due to malingering or hysteria. While malingering implies the willful feigning or exaggeration of symptoms, and hysteria suggests a subconscious expression of the nonorganic signs or symptoms, differentiation of the two functional types, other than through observation of visual behavior when the patient is unaware of surveillance, is extremely difficult, even for psychiatric experts.

Patients with hysterical neuro-ophthalmic complaints have little or no insight into their infirmity, and they display a singular lack of concern over their quite incapacitating symptoms (*la belle indifférence*). The malingering patient usually can be found to have some type of primary gain for the infirmity and may even come to the examination with an attitude defying the examiner to uncover the ailment.

Although we consider the distinction between hysteria and malingering to be extremely important in the treatment of these individuals, a clear separation may not be possible.

The most common presentations of functional visual loss are constricted fields or decreased acuity in one or both eyes.

Additional Testing

No testing beyond the clinical and visual field examination of the patient should be required. Pattern-shift visually evoked potentials may help substantiate the normalcy of the afferent visual pathways, but the wary patient may fixate beyond the pattern stimuli, obliterating the P_{100} response and further confusing the picture. It should, however, be remembered that some individuals with true organic disease will add on a large degree of functional overlay, and that a casual diagnosis of purely functional disease may overlook a potentially serious disease. This diagnosis should, therefore, be made only after careful documentation of the mismatch of objective and subjective findings. If there is any question as to the authenticity of the patient's objective and subjective findings, neuro-imaging studies of the appropriate areas should be obtained.

Treatment

The treatment of the patient with functional visual loss is often an experiment in frustration. In the malingering patient it is important to document carefully the findings supporting the nonexistence of an organic problem, and then give the patient a way out of this predicament by suggesting that if he or she does in fact "have a problem," it is one that will improve over time. Then the clinician should follow the patient to ensure that he or she will not further abuse the medical care system. Patients often accept eagerly a way to "save face" if the alternative is humiliation from exposure of the fraud to relatives and friends.

In the patient with hysterical visual field constriction, therapy should be directed toward the primary psychiatric disorder. This is often beyond the means of the nonpsychiatric clinician.

Management and Course of the Case

The patient was referred for psychotherapy regarding her inability to cope with the death of the pedestrian as a result of her accident. Within 3 months her visual deficit had resolved entirely.

Monocular Functional Visual Loss

A 27-year-old software engineer complained of an inability to see his work after having had a chemical inadvertently splashed into his left eye by a fellow employee. He had been seen immediately after the accident in a local emergency room where his eye was noted to be red with "poor vision." He appeared for the examination demanding to be compensated for the loss of his ability to carry out his rigorous duties. Visual acuity was 20/20 on the right and no light perception on the left with symmetrically reactive pupils and no relative afferent pupillary defect. Perimetry was performed with both eyes open.

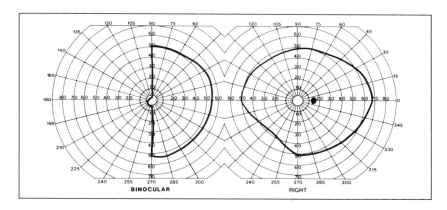

The binocular visual field is clearly nonanatomic with an abrupt cutoff of field at the midline and a normal monocular right field. The presence of normal pupillary reactions is further supportive evidence that both afferent visual systems are functioning normally. When it was suggested that his visual infirmity was one that would improve and that he should be able to continue working, the patient angrily left the office.

Other testing helpful in the presence of claimed (but suspected functional) monocular blindness is the optokinetic nystagmus (OKN) response, stereopsis, the prism shift test, and pattern-shift evoked potentials.

The presence of a monocular response to the moving OKN strip (or to a moving mirror that is placed in front of a patient with one eye covered) suggests that visual input is being transmitted and is inconsistent with claimed monocular blindness. If the OKN strip (or drum) is then moved to a distance of 10 feet, the continued presence of a monocular response implies an acuity of better than 20/100. This is a very helpful test, therefore, for claimed monocular blindness or markedly reduced acuity.

The presence of stereopsis indicates binocularity. If the patient can identify all dots on the Titmus stereo test, the visual acuity can be established as at least 20/30 in each eye—an assessment more refined than the considerably more expensive evoked potential testing! In addition, a stereoscopic visual acuity chart may be used. With this test each eye sees different letters unbeknownst to the patient. Red-green letters can also be used for this purpose, but the patient will often catch on and not read letters with his "bad" eye.

The prism shift test is performed as follows: As the patient fixates on a letter on a Snellen's chart requiring 20/40 or better acuity, a 4-diopter base-out prism is introduced in front of the "bad" eye. If a compensatory shift to regain binocular fixation on the target is observed, then it can be assumed that the purported poor-sighted eye was seeing at that particular level of acuity. A vertical prism can also be placed in front of one eye while the patient is reading the eye chart binocularly. This will separate the vision in the two eyes such that two lines of letters are seen. If the patient reports seeing the doubled letters then he or she must be seeing well out of both eyes.

In monocular functional vision loss the comparison of objective responses between eyes makes testing for functional disease much easier than in binocular functional visual complaints, in which the technique of perimetry may be more difficult and lack of objective evidence for afferent visual system dysfunction harder to demonstrate. A mismatch of findings on the afferent visual system exam with the patient's claimed subjective complaints should, however, be the clue to the presence of functional disease, either binocular or monocular.

Bibliography

Bumgartner, J., and Epstein, C. M. Voluntary alteration of visual evoked potentials. *Ann. Neurol.* 12:475, 1982.

Chiappa, K. H., and Yiannikas, C. Voluntary alteration of evoked potential? *Ann. Neurol.* 12:496, 1982.

Kathol, R. G., et al. Functional visual loss: Follow-up of 42 cases. *Arch. Ophthalmol.* 101:729, 1983.

Keane, J. R. Neuro-ophthalmic signs and symptoms of hysteria. *Neurology* 32:757, 1982.

Keltner, J. L., et al. The California syndrome: Functional vision complaints with potential economic impact. *Ophthalmology* 92:427, 1985.

Kramer, K. K., La Piana, F. G., and Appleton, B. Ocular malingering and hysteria: Diagnosis and management. *Surv. Ophthalmol.* 24:89, 1979.

Smith, C. H., Beck, R. W., and Mills, R. P. Functional disease in neuro-ophthalmology. *Neurol. Clin.* 1:955, 1983.

Thompson, H. S. Functional visual loss. *Am. J. Ophthalmol.* 100:209, 1985.

22

Limited Upgaze— Graves' Ophthalmopathy

A 32-year-old man was examined because of intermittent vertical diplopia present for 1 year. The diplopia had worsened (increased in frequency) over the initial several months but had been stable for the 2 months before examination. It was at its worse on awakening in the morning. He was otherwise in good health with no medical problems or medications.

Neuro-Ophthalmic Examination

	OD	OS
Visual acuity	20/20	20/20
Pupils	Normal	Normal
Lid apertures	11 mm	11 mm
Exophthalmometry findings	18 mm	17 mm
Visual field	Normal	Normal
Fundi	Normal	Normal

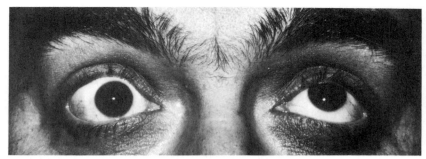

Upgaze

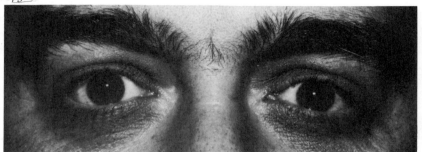

Primary position

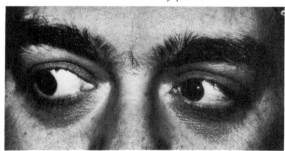

Right gaze

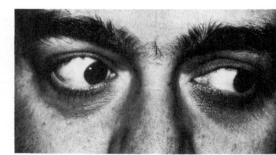

Left gaze

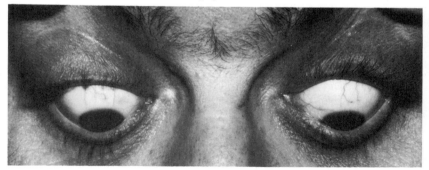

Downgaze

The patient had a 12-prism-diopter left hypertropia (right hypotropia) in the primary position but could fuse with slight chin elevation. There was no deviation in downgaze.

Summary

A 32-year-old man with 1 year of intermittent diplopia was found to have limitation of upgaze in the right eye.

Differential Diagnosis

Motility testing demonstrated that the patient's diplopia was due to limitation of upgaze of the right eye. The Bielschowsky three-step test is not necessary nor usually helpful when there is an obvious limitation of gaze.

The major causes of limited upgaze that should be considered include (1) restriction of the inferior rectus, most commonly secondary to inflammation (Graves' disease, myositis) or a blowout fracture; (2) partial third nerve palsy; and (3) myasthenia gravis. Any of these would be a possible cause in this patient. Graves' ophthalmopathy commonly affects the inferior rectus. If lid retraction is present in association with a vertical ophthalmoplegia (although not present in this case), Graves' is almost always the diagnosis. A partial third nerve palsy usually does not affect just one muscle, but isolated involvement of a muscle, particularly the superior rectus, is possible. Ptosis often accompanies the superior rectus involvement, but this is not invariable (see Limited Upgaze—Third Nerve Palsy from Cavernous Sinus Mass, below). Myasthenia gravis can cause any type of pupil-sparing motility disorder. Although there is usually evidence of involvement of the levator or multiple extraocular muscles, it is possible for a patient to have apparent abnormality restricted to one muscle.

Less common causes of a unilateral limitation of upgaze include congenital double elevator palsy, Brown's superior oblique tendon sheath syndrome, orbital tumors, underaction of a contralateral antagonist muscle (the contralateral superior rectus in a superior oblique palsy), a brainstem lesion, and a myopathy. In the first two entities there will usually be a history of a motility disorder since childhood. A brainstem lesion could rarely produce a unilateral upgaze palsy, but virtually always other brainstem signs will be present and will usually predominate, leaving little difficulty in diagnosis. A myopathy would be expected to produce abnormalities in multiple muscles in both eyes.

Additional testing is necessary to establish a diagnosis. A forced duction test should be performed. A positive result (demonstrating limitation) would suggest inferior rectus restriction as the primary cause of the impairment in upgaze, but in any long-standing paretic process, the forced duction test may have a positive result. If the forced duction test has a negative result, a Tensilon test should be performed. If diagnosis remains in doubt, a computed tomography (CT) or magnetic resonance imaging scan will be necessary to determine whether there is an orbital or intracranial cause.

In this case a forced duction test had positive results. CT demonstrated the presence of an enlarged right inferior rectus muscle (see p. 156). Thyroid function tests showed an elevated T_4 and T_3 and a low TSH.

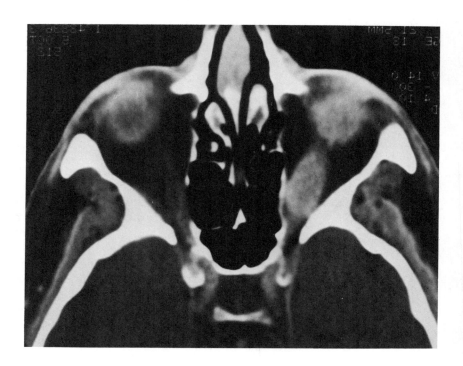

Clinical Diagnosis: Graves' Ophthalmopathy

Graves' disease is an immune-mediated disorder characterized by hyperthyroidism with diffuse hyperplasia of the thyroid gland, pretibial myxedema, and ophthalmopathy. There is not a direct cause-effect relationship between the thyroid disease and eye muscle involvement. In fact at the time of eye involvement there may be no past or current overt or serologic evidence of thyroid disease (euthyroid Graves' disease).

The ophthalmopathy may develop at any age. Females are affected more often than males. Presenting symptoms and signs vary considerably in the disease. The American Thyroid Association has adopted a seven-stage classification of the eye changes in Graves' disease: 0—no symptoms or signs; 1—lid signs; 2—soft tissue changes; 3—proptosis; 4—extraocular muscle involvement; 5—corneal changes; 6—optic neuropathy. Although this scheme may be useful in categorizing a patient's findings, it is of little value in staging a given patient's disease since there is frequently not a natural progression from one class to the next. It is more useful to specify separately the changes related to involvement of the conjunctiva (injection, chemosis), cornea (epithelial defects), eyelids (swelling, lid retraction), extraocular muscles (diplopia), and optic nerve (visual loss).

Diplopia is the most common disabling symptom of Graves' disease. With inflammation of an extraocular muscle, it becomes less elastic and restricts the movement of the eye in the direction of gaze opposite the muscle. This change can be confirmed with a forced duction test (see Chapter 1). Histopathologically the muscles show a perivascular mononuclear cell infiltration, interstitial edema, and an increase in mucopolysaccharides during the active phase and later fibrosis. Any pattern of extraocular muscle involvement is possible. The inferior rectus and medial rectus muscles are involved more commonly than the superior or lateral recti.

Optic nerve involvement is the most dreaded complication of Graves' ophthalmopathy since irreversible blindness is possible. This occurrence is described in detail in Chapter 16.

Diagnosis of Graves' disease as a cause of diplopia or optic neuropathy can usually be made on clinical grounds. Orbital and lid signs can be very helpful in diagnosis but are not always present. Proptosis may be unilateral or bilateral, but in some cases, even when extraocular muscle involvement is marked, proptosis is not apparent. The reason for this is not known. The diagnosis of Graves' disease as a cause of ophthalmoplegia is all too often missed when proptosis is absent. Lid retraction may occur from mechanical restriction of the levator muscle caused by fibrosis similar to the extraocular muscle involvement. In association with proptosis and ophthalmoplegia, lid retraction is virtually pathognomonic of Graves' disease.

Additional Testing

In patients with a history of thyroid disease and classic eye signs, no additional studies are necessary other than assuring that the patient is euthyroid. With no history of thyroid disease, thyroid blood tests should be performed. CT scanning or orbital ultrasound is not necessary in all cases. If no thyroid dysfunction is identified by history or blood tests or if the ocular changes are not completely typical for Graves' ophthalmopathy, then orbital imaging is important to confirm the diagnosis. In obvious cases it is superfluous. CT changes are usually confined to the muscles. Classically, the belly of the muscle is enlarged and the tendon portion appears normal.

Treatment

Graves' ophthalmopathy is a self-limited disorder that remains active in most patients for a period lasting from a few months to two to three years. Although there is no therapy for the disease itself, many of the complications of the disease can be effectively treated.

External symptoms of dryness and grittiness can be treated with artificial tear preparations and methylcellulose ointments. When lid retraction is marked, surgical correction is warranted once the disease has remained quiescent for at least 6 months. Corticosteroids are generally not indicated for the soft tissue changes, but an occasional patient will have marked soft tissue inflammation that may warrant steroid use. Radiation therapy for symptomatic relief should be considered only in rare severe cases.

Diplopia is the most common disabling symptom requiring treatment. Initial treatment usually consists of patching one eye or occasionally prescribing a prism. Corticosteroids may be considered if the ocular deviation is small and of recent onset but should not be used chronically. Muscle surgery is the mainstay of therapy but should be deferred until the disease has been quiescent and the ocular deviation stable for at least 6 months. Surgery generally consists of recession on adjustable sutures of the muscles most responsible for the deviation. Radiation is usually not effective in alleviating diplopia.

The treatment of the optic neuropathy is discussed in Chapter 16.

Management and Course of the Case

The patient received treatment with radioactive I_{131} for the hyperthyroidism. By assuming a head position with slight chin elevation, he minimized diplopia. Since he was only minimally symptomatic from the diplopia, no treatment was prescribed. His condition has remained unchanged in 2 years of follow-up.

Limited Upgaze—Third Nerve Palsy from Cavernous Sinus Mass

A 57-year-old woman noted diplopia when looking over her shoulder to back out her car for 1 year. She had no symptoms at other times.

On examination she had limitation of upgaze in the left eye but otherwise full motility. There were no lid or orbital signs.

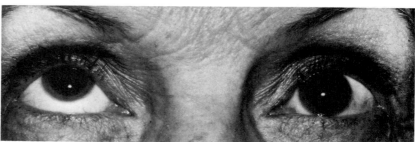

Upgaze

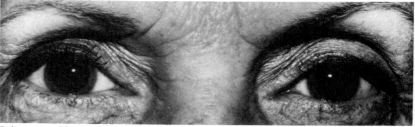

Primary position

Results of a forced duction test were positive. Thyroid function studies had normal results. A CT scan demonstrated a mass in the region of the left cavernous sinus.

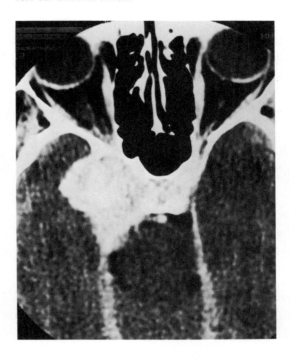

The mass seen on CT was presumed to be a meningioma, but because the patient was only minimally symptomatic, no further studies or procedures were performed. Her condition has remained unchanged in 2 years of follow-up.

Although Graves' disease was initially contemplated as the diagnosis, since there were no lid or orbital signs and no evidence of thyroid dysfunction, the CT scan was performed. Although additional evidence of third nerve involvement would be expected with a tumor this size, we have seen isolated superior rectus paresis in several other cases of cavernous sinus lesions. The positive result of the forced duction test in this case was the result of secondary contracture of the inferior rectus and not indicative of a primary restrictive process.

Limited Upgaze from Blowout Fracture

A 15-year-old boy suffered facial trauma in a motor vehicle accident. The photographs below demonstrate limitation of upgaze in the left eye. Results of a forced duction test were positive, and a diagnosis of blowout fracture was made and confirmed by tomography. A surgical repair was performed.

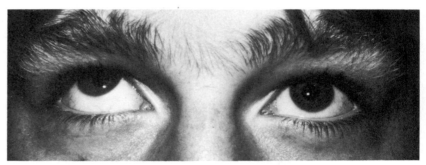

Upgaze

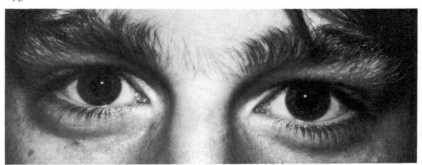

Primary position

Limited Upgaze from Myasthenia Gravis

A 70-year-old man was examined 2 days after the onset of diplopia. He was otherwise well and had noted no other problems.

His examination was remarkable for right ptosis (which he had not noted) and limitation of upgaze in the right eye. He had a 4-prism-diopter left hypertropia in the primary position and a 12-diopter left hypertropia in upgaze.

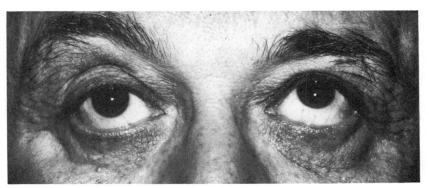

Upgaze

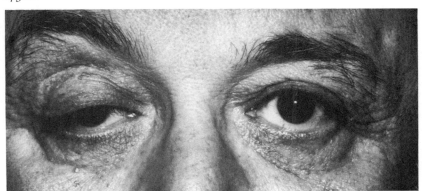

Primary position

Initially a superior division third nerve palsy was suspected. A CT scan was normal. A Tensilon test was then performed with complete resolution of the ptosis and hypertropia. A diagnosis of myasthenia gravis was made. This case illustrates how myasthenia can mimic a motility disorder that is consistent with a neurogenic cause.

Bibliography

Brennan, M. W., Leone, C. R., and Janaki, L. Radiation therapy for Graves' disease. *Am. J. Ophthalmol.* 96:195, 1983.

Evans, D., and Kennerdell, J. S. Extraocular muscle surgery for dysthyroid myopathy. *Am. J. Ophthalmol.* 95:767, 1983.

Felberg, N. T., et al. Lymphocyte subpopulations in Graves' ophthalmopathy. *Arch. Ophthalmol.* 103:656, 1985.

Feldon, S. E., and Weiner, J. M. Clinical significance of extraocular muscle volumes in Graves' ophthalmopathy. *Arch. Ophthalmol.* 100:1266, 1982.

Hufnagel, T. J., et al. Immunohistochemical and ultrastructural studies on the exenterated orbital tissues of a patient with Graves' disease. *Ophthalmology* 91:1411, 1984.

Hurbli, T., et al. Radiation therapy for thyroid eye diseases. *Am. J. Ophthalmol.* 99:633, 1985.

Jacobson, D. H., and Gorman, C. A. Endocrine ophthalmopathy: Current ideas concerning etiology, pathogenesis, and treatment. *Endocr. Rev.* 5:200, 1984.

Leone, C. R. The management of ophthalmic Graves' disease. *Ophthalmology* 91:770, 1984.

Sergott, R. C., and Glaser, J. S. Graves' ophthalmopathy: A clinical and immunologic review. *Surv. Ophthalmol.* 26:1, 1981.

Uretsky, S. H., Kennerdell, J. S., and Gutai, J. P. Graves' ophthalmopathy in childhood and adolescence. *Arch. Ophthalmol.* 98:1963, 1980.

23

Fourth Nerve Palsy

A 76-year-old man reported the sudden onset of diplopia. There were no associated symptoms. He was otherwise in good health. His medical history was notable only for medically controlled hypertension.

Neuro-Ophthalmic Examination

	OD	OS
Visual acuity	20/20	20/20
Pupils	Normal	Normal
Lids, orbits	Normal	Normal
Motility	Full	Full
Visual field	Full	Full
Fundi	Normal	Normal

Three-Step Test

1. Primary position — 3-prism-diopter (PD) right hypertropia
2. Right gaze — Orthophoric
   Left gaze — 9-PD right hypertropia
3. Right head tilt — 12-PD right hypertropia
   Left head tilt — 2-PD right hypertropia

Summary
A 76-year-old man with recent onset of diplopia was found to have a right hypertropia that was greater on left gaze and right head tilt.

Differential Diagnosis
The three-step test identified the diplopia as a superior oblique palsy. The performance and interpretation of the three-step test are detailed in Chapter 1. Causes of a superior oblique palsy are discussed below.

Clinical Diagnosis: Superior Oblique Palsy

A superior oblique palsy is a common cause of acquired vertical diplopia. The trochlear nerve innervates the superior oblique muscle from the contralateral side of the brainstem. Following their exit dorsally from the brainstem, the trochlear nerves cross in the anterior medullary velum and then proceed forward, crossing the superior cerebellar arteries before piercing the dura and entering the cavernous sinuses. The nerve can be damaged anywhere along its course. Without evidence of other neurologic involvement, localization is not possible.

The most common cause of a trochlear nerve palsy is head trauma— usually severe head trauma with loss of consciousness present. Minor head injuries producing a palsy suggest the possibility of a tumor that has tethered the nerve, making it more susceptible to injury. The trochlear nerve may be damaged as it exits the brainstem, crosses in the anterior medullary velum, or passes through the superior orbital fissure. Bilateral fourth nerve palsies following trauma are not uncommon and presumably occur where the two nerves cross in the anterior medullary velum. The prognosis for recovery of a traumatic fourth nerve palsy is good. More than 50 percent of the time there is complete resolution.

In the patient without a history of trauma, there are several etiologic considerations. In seeking a cause it is important to determine whether the fourth nerve palsy is an isolated finding or whether there are other neurologic abnormalities. With brainstem lesions other neurologic deficits usually predominate and allow localization of the problem. Isolated fourth nerve palsies in patients older than 50 are usually due to microvascular ischemia. Onset is typically sudden, and resolution over several months occurs in most patients. A postviral syndrome is the most common cause in a child, as it is for the other ocular motor nerve palsies. Compressive lesions uncommonly produce isolated fourth nerve palsies, but rarely a posterior fossa tumor or aneurysm, especially of the superior cerebellar artery, is the cause. Although a cavernous sinus lesion usually affects multiple nerves, it can impair just one nerve, and an isolated fourth nerve palsy would be possible.

Not infrequently a fourth nerve palsy presenting in adulthood, especially in patients between 20 and 40, is the result of the breakdown of a congenital palsy. This is diagnosed by the presence of a larger than normal vertical fusional amplitude, history of intermittent diplopia when tired or ill in the past, and head tilt on old photographs. The normal vertical fusional amplitude is only about 3 prism diopters. Patients with a breakdown of a congenital palsy often have amplitudes of 10 diopters or greater. Presentation does not occur until adulthood because the fusional amplitude gradually decreases as the patient gets older and reaches a point at which it is too small to control the tendency for the eyes to separate.

As has been mentioned throughout this text, myasthenia gravis must be considered as the potential cause of any ophthalmoplegia, and a superior oblique palsy is no exception.

Diagnosis of a fourth nerve palsy is made on the three-step test as noted above. Often the weakness of the superior oblique muscle on motility testing will not be very apparent. With a unilateral fourth nerve palsy, there is generally a hypertropia of from 3 to 15 diopters and an excyclodeviation of 5 to 10 degrees. A small esotropia may also be noted, particularly in downgaze. Bilateral fourth nerve palsies, which are not uncommon after head injuries, usually produce little deviation in the primary position. A right hypertropia is present on left gaze and right head tilt; a left hypertropia is present on right gaze and left head tilt. Often one of the nerves will be impaired more than the other, and not infrequently the bilaterality of the problem will not be appreciated by the physician. An excyclodeviation of greater than 15 degrees or a V-pattern esotropia of greater than 25 diopters from upgaze to downgaze is strongly suggestive of bilateral palsies.

In all patients (without a history of head trauma) the possibility of the diplopia being the result of the breakdown of a congenital palsy should be considered. Fusional amplitudes should be measured and when appropriate old photographs viewed. Otherwise, the workup of an isolated nontraumatic fourth nerve palsy depends on the age of the patient. In a patient older than 50, the workup can be limited to a general physical examination and an evaluation for risk factors for vascular disease—hypertension, diabetes, elevation of cholesterol and triglycerides. Should the palsy be progressive or not improving within 3 months, a computed tomography (CT) or magnetic resonance imaging (MRI) scan should be performed. In a child with a recent history of a viral infection, observation is prudent. Again, should the course become atypical or other signs develop, a neuroradiologic evaluation is necessary. In patients between the ages of 10 and 50 in whom there is no indication that the palsy is congenital, a more complete investigation should be performed. These patients should be evaluated for hypertension, diabetes, and vasculitis and a CT or MRI scan should be performed. If all of these tests have normal results, a lumbar puncture may be considered. In all age groups, a Tensilon test should be performed whenever diagnosis is in doubt.

Treatment

Most fourth nerve palsies improve in time, so treatment for the most part is a temporizing measure. Often the patient will alleviate the diplopia by head posturing—turning and tilting the head to the side opposite the palsy and depressing the chin. If diplopia remains a problem, however, then it is prudent to cover one eye or try a Fresnel prism.

Surgical correction should not be considered for at least 6 months from the time of onset of the palsy. If there has been no improvement by that time, it is not likely to occur. Weakening procedures on the inferior oblique muscle and strengthening procedures on the superior oblique both have a role.

Management and Course of the Case

Blood pressure was 140/85. Serum glucose, cholesterol, and triglyceride levels were normal. Results of a general physical examination were unremarkable. A cover was placed on one lens of the patient's glasses. He was examined again after 2 weeks, and there was no change in his measurements. At 6 weeks his diplopia had improved and was present only in left gaze, where it measured 4 diopters. At 3 months he was asymptomatic, and the hypertropia had resolved.

Bilateral Fourth Nerve Palsies

A 24-year-old man noted diplopia after a head injury suffered in a motor vehicle accident that produced loss of consciousness for 12 hours.

On motility testing limitation of downgaze in the adducted position was noted in the right eye. Range of motion was otherwise full.

His measurements were as follows:

1. Primary position	2-PD right hypertropia
2. Right gaze	2-PD left hypertropia
Left gaze	12-PD right hypertropia
3. Right head tilt	14-PD right hypertropia
Left head tilt	3-PD left hypertropia
4. Excyclodeviation	15 degrees

The measurements in this case indicate the patient has bilateral fourth nerve palsies. Although involvement is asymmetric, the findings of the left hypertropia on gaze right and left head tilt indicate that the left fourth nerve is involved in addition to the right. The magnitude of the excyclodeviation is larger than usually seen with a unilateral palsy and also suggests the bilaterality.

Congenital Fourth Nerve Palsy

A 21-year-old man was examined because of headaches and diplopia. The headaches had been recurrent for several years and were consistent with common migraine. Diplopia had occurred intermittently for the previous 6 months, mainly late in the day when he was tired. During his most recent migraine, diplopia had been present for several hours.

On examination he had a 14-prism-diopter right hyperphoria, which increased on left gaze and right head tilt. Vertical fusional amplitude was 20 prism diopters. Old photographs showed a slight head tilt to the left.

The results of the three-step test were diagnostic of a fourth nerve palsy. The large fusional amplitude and the presence of the head tilt on the old photographs were most consistent with a congenital cause for the palsy. The fact that the deviation was a phoria and not a tropia by itself indicated that fusional amplitudes were larger than normal. Diplopia occurred when he was tired or during the headache because his fusional amplitude decreased at those times.

Bibliography

Ellis, F. D., and Helveston, E. M. Superior oblique palsy: Diagnosis and classification. *Int. Ophthalmol. Clin.* 16 (3): 127, 1976.

Lee, J., and Flynn, J. T. Bilateral superior oblique palsies. *Br. J. Ophthalmol.* 69: 508, 1985.

Rush, J. A., and Younge, B. R. Paralysis of cranial nerves III, IV and VI. *Arch. Ophthalmol.* 99: 76, 1981.

Sydnor, C. F., Seaber, J. H., and Buckley, E. G. Traumatic superior oblique palsies. *Ophthalmology* 89: 134, 1982.

Younge, B. R., and Sutula, F. Analysis of trochlear nerve palsies. *Mayo Clin. Proc.* 52: 11, 1977.

24

Third Nerve Palsy

A 79-year-old woman had a 4-week history of unrelenting right retro-orbital pain. She had been seen by a neurologist 1 week previously and had been found to have normal examination results and a normal head computed tomography (CT) scan. During the 3 days before her admission to the hospital she began complaining of horizontal diplopia and a droopy right eyelid.

Neuro-Ophthalmic Examination

	OD	OS
Visual acuity	20/20	20/20
Color plates correct	12 of 12	12 of 12
Pupils	7 mm and fixed	3 mm and brisk
Motility and lids	See below	
Orbits	Normal	Normal
Visual field	Normal	Normal
Fundi	Normal	Normal

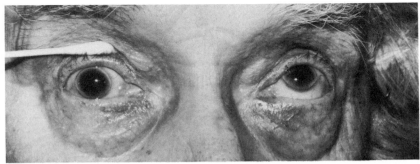

Upgaze

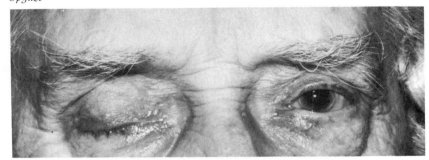

Primary position

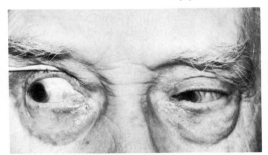

Right gaze

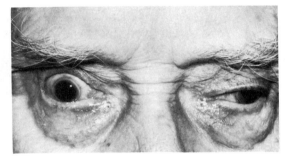

Left gaze

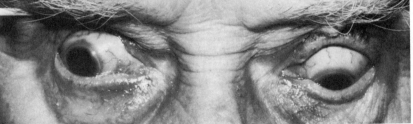

Downgaze

Summary
A 79-year-old woman with a painful ophthalmoplegia, dilated pupil, and ptosis in the right eye was found to have a normal CT scan.

Differential Diagnosis

Adduction deficits associated with ptosis and pupillary involvement localize the lesion to the oculomotor (third) nerve. Ptosis is rarely seen in association with a restrictive orbitopathy. The presence of a fixed dilated pupil rules out myasthenia as a consideration. If the pupil had not been involved, a forced duction test and Tensilon testing would have been necessary to rule out the latter two possibilities.

The majority of patients presenting with retro-orbital pain and isolated third nerve paresis of acute or subacute onset will have either an aneurysm compressing the third nerve or an infarction involving the nerve parenchyma. Less common causes include tumor compression, uncal herniation syndrome, migraine, vasculitis, trauma, and meningitis.

The real issue facing the clinician in this case is whether the presenting signs indicate an ischemic process to the third nerve that will improve with observation, or whether they mandate immediate arteriography to visualize a potentially curable but life-threatening aneurysm. In this patient dilation of the pupil is highly suggestive of an aneurysm or other compressive lesion.

Clinical Diagnosis: Third Nerve Palsy, Probable Aneurysm

The third cranial nerve exits the midbrain ventrally to enter the cavernous sinus after passing adjacent to the tentorial edge. The parasympathetic fibers accompany the third nerve and supply input to the pupil and ciliary body. In the cavernous sinus the third nerve lies in proximity to the fourth, sixth, fifth (first division), and sympathetic nerves. It then enters the orbit through the superior orbital fissure to supply four extraocular muscles and the levator of the lid. Lesions involving the third nerve can be grouped anatomically into nuclear, fascicular, subarachnoid, tentorial edge, cavernous sinus, and orbital types; the more common causes in these regions are outlined in Table 24-1.

In general, compressive lesions of the third nerve can be localized by the appearance of contiguous neurologic findings in the anatomic subgroups outlined. The major differentiating points between an ischemic and compressive third nerve paresis are outlined in Table 24-2.

The major clinical findings that help differentiate between compressive and ischemic third nerve paresis are the presence of pain, aberrant regeneration, and pupillary involvement.

The pain present with ischemia of the third nerve parenchyma is usually mild and clears within days. Pain from aneurysmal compression of the third nerve is typically severe and is relieved only with nerve decompression.

Aberrant regeneration of the third nerve may be characterized by lid retraction or pupillary constriction in attempted downgaze ("pseudo–von Graefe phenomenon") or adduction. The mechanism for the aberrant movements is not known, but it appears to be either the aberrant regrowth of axons after disruption of the axon cylinders or third nerve

Table 24-1. Causes of third nerve palsy

Nuclear
   Congenital
   Vascular insult
   Trauma
   Migraine*
Fascicular
   Compressive lesion
   Ischemic
   Vasculitis
   Trauma
Subarachnoid
   Compressive (aneurysm, tumor)
   Meningitis
   Vascular (ischemic)
   Trauma
Tentorial edge
   Uncal herniation
   Trauma
Cavernous sinus
   Aneurysm
   Tumor (meningioma, pituitary adenoma, metastatic)
   Pituitary apoplexy (see Chapter 17)
   Vascular (ischemic)
   Inflammatory (Tolosa-Hunt syndrome; see Chapter 30)
Orbital
   Trauma
   Vascular (arteritis, ischemic)

*Location of lesion uncertain.

nuclear reorganization at a brainstem level. Aberrant regeneration may be seen with any compressive or traumatic lesion of the third nerve. Its appearance without a history of acute oculomotor palsy should suggest a lesion involving the cavernous sinus region. Aberrant regeneration has also been seen transiently after ophthalmoplegic migraine. It is not a feature of ischemic third nerve paresis.

The pupillary fibers travel superficially and superonasally in the third nerve, which leaves them more susceptible to external compression than to the effects of an intrinsic nerve lesion from vascular infarction. The concept of *pupil sparing* is frequently misunderstood. If a pupil is at all larger than its fellow, or not normally reactive, then it should be considered involved. Physiologic anisocoria can easily be distinguished from a

Table 24-2. Ischemic versus compressive third nerve paresis

Feature	Ischemic	Compressive
Associated signs	Infrequent	Usually present
Pain	Variable	Usually present
Pupillary involvement	5%	95%
Aberrant regeneration	Not seen	Seen with chronic compressive lesions
Age at onset	Late adulthood	Any age

pathologic pupillary dilation, because in the former the difference in diameters between the two pupils does not change with a change in ambient lighting (see Chapter 34). Although 8 to 15 percent of those with third nerve palsies caused by aneurysms have been reported to have temporary or initial pupillary sparing, complete pupillary sparing at the time of presentation with an aneurysm is rare.

Of the compressive lesions leading to a third nerve palsy, aneurysm and tumor are the most common. With the standard enhanced CT scan, a mass lesion outside the cavernous sinus can be excluded. An aneurysm involving the posterior communicating artery may not show up even on a good CT scan; this diagnosis can be excluded only after either conventional cerebral angiography or high-quality intraarterial digital subtraction angiography has been carried out. The acute or subacute onset of a pupil-involving third nerve palsy should always suggest the diagnosis of an aneurysm—even when a CT scan has been found to be normal.

Additional Testing

When pupillary involvement is seen with a third nerve paresis, the patient should be admitted to the hospital immediately and either a CT scan or a magnetic resonance imaging scan should be performed to check for a mass lesion. If these studies are normal (or not definitive), four-vessel conventional or digital (intraarterial) cerebral angiography should be performed to look for an aneurysm. If all of these studies have normal results a lumbar puncture is necessary to rule out meningitis.

The diabetic or hypertensive older patient with a pupil-sparing third nerve paresis should be examined to ensure that the primary disease process (diabetes or hypertension) has been adequately controlled. An erythrocyte sedimentation rate (ESR) should be obtained to check for giant cell arteritis, and the patient should be followed weekly for several weeks. In this group of patients, no neuroimaging studies are obtained unless there is progression of the palsy or additional signs develop.

In the patient with a pupil-sparing third nerve paresis and no obvious vascular explanation for an ischemic insult, a fasting blood sugar level, an ESR, an antinuclear antibody test, and careful blood pressure readings should be obtained to check for diabetes, systemic vasculitis, syphilis, and hypertension. Neuroimaging studies are obtained in this group on an individual basis. The patient should be examined daily during the first week after the onset of the palsy for signs of pupillary involvement and thereafter every 1 or 2 weeks until the palsy starts to show improvement.

Management and Course of the Case

An arteriogram confirmed the presence of an aneurysm, which originated from the internal carotid artery just before the takeoff of the posterior communicating artery. The aneurysm was clipped without in-

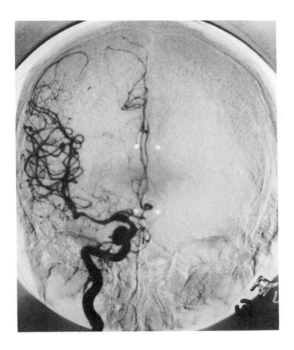

cident, and her diplopia and ptosis have cleared entirely. After 1 year of follow-up her right pupil remains poorly responsive to light.

Third Nerve Palsy—Ischemia

A 63-year-old man was referred for evaluation of complete right ptosis and diplopia of abrupt onset. He had had mild right retro-orbital pain for the 24 hours preceding the onset of the ptosis. He had mild adult-onset diabetes and 5 years previously had had a left carotid arteriogram for transient ischemic attack symptoms. He had a complete right ptosis with the right eye externally rotated and slightly down. There was limitation of upgaze, downgaze, and adduction in the right eye. The right pupil was 2 mm greater than the left (3 mm greater in dim lighting) and reacted normally to light. The only other abnormal finding on examination was mild diabetic retinopathy.

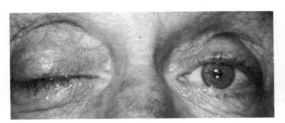
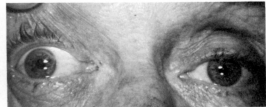

With lid held

This patient has a pupil-sparing right third nerve palsy with an old left Horner's syndrome (see Chapter 33), which was confirmed by old photographs and cocaine testing. The Horner's syndrome was presumed to be the result of the direct puncture carotid arteriogram he had had previously.

The third nerve palsy was thought to be secondary to microvascular ischemia, and the patient was observed without neuroimaging studies. His third nerve paresis cleared without residua. The left Horner's syndrome persisted.

Third Nerve Palsy—Aberrant Regeneration

A 33-year-old man noted the progressive onset of diplopia and right-sided ptosis associated with a tingling feeling over the right supraorbital region. His examination showed normal acuity, visual fields, and color vision; general neurologic examination also had normal results. There was limitation of upgaze and adduction in the right eye. The right upper lid, which was ptotic in the primary position, elevated on adduction (see below). Downgaze was normal.

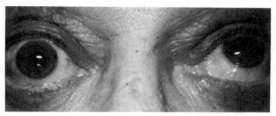

Upgaze

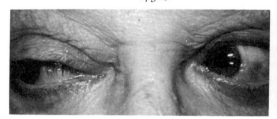

Right gaze

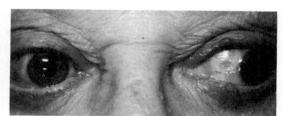

Left gaze

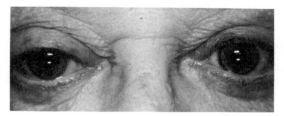

Primary position

CT scan demonstrated an intra-cavernous-sinus mass extending into the middle fossa on the right. The arteriogram was consistent with mass effect in this region. Biopsy of this mass confirmed the presence of a meningioma. The patient elected to have no further therapy; his condition has remained stable over a 3-year period.

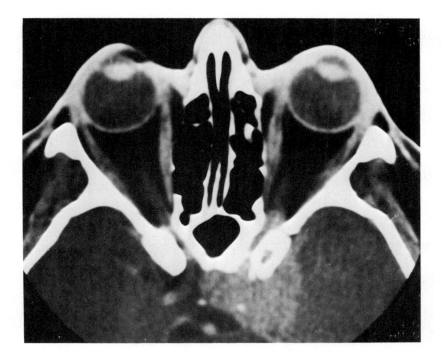

Lid elevation on adduction or on downgaze in the presence of a partial third nerve paresis suggests aberrant regeneration. The symptom of supraorbital dysesthesias suggests involvement of the first division of the trigeminal nerve, which further localizes the lesion to the cavernous sinus. The absence of proptosis or other orbital findings suggests a compressive lesion in the region of the cavernous sinus. Aberrant regeneration of the third nerve without history of acute oculomotor palsy is seen most commonly in patients with cavernous sinus compressive lesions.

Tumors within the cavernous sinus cannot be removed surgically and are not particularly radiosensitive. Meningiomas are generally benign, slow-growing tumors that create morbidity by their pressure effect as they expand. In this case the only reason to operate was to determine the histologic type of the tumor and debulk it if it were causing intra-cranial damage from its extension outside the cavernous sinus.

Third Nerve Palsy from Cavernous Sinus Aneurysm

A 53-year-old woman noted left orbital pain and diplopia that progressively worsened over a 1-year period. For the previous 2 months she had had a sensation of "pins and needles" over the left eyebrow region. Visual acuity was 20/20 in each eye with normal fundi and full visual fields. She had mild right ptosis with limitation of elevation, adduction, and depression of the right eye.

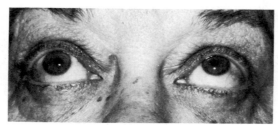

Upgaze

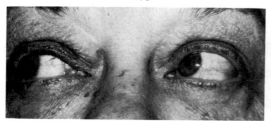

Right gaze

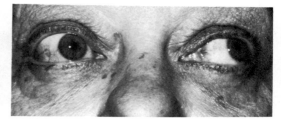

Left gaze

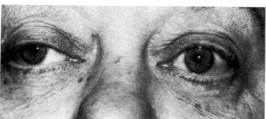

Primary position

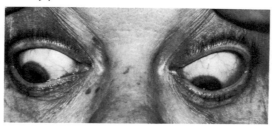

Downgaze

This third nerve paresis was associated with symptoms of trigeminal (first division) irritation, which suggested involvement of the cavernous sinus. The CT scan confirmed the presence of bilateral cavernous sinus masses with a calcified rim—apparently intra-cavernous sinus aneurysms. This was confirmed on a cerebral angiogram. No surgical correction was attempted, and her findings have remained unchanged for the past 2 years.

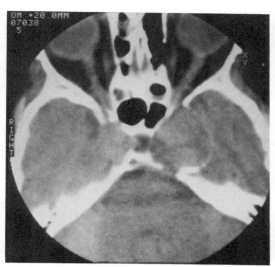

Without contrast

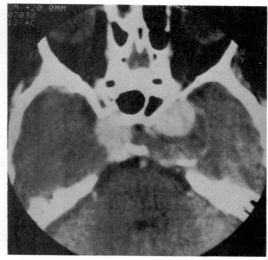

With contrast

Intra-cavernous sinus aneurysms may cause considerable pain in addition to a cavernous sinus syndrome, but they rarely hemorrhage or are fatal. However, the various surgical methods of correcting an aneurysm situated in this area may lead to major morbidity or even death. Therefore we recommend a surgical approach only if the patient is incapacitated by pain and fully understands the treatment options.

Bibliography

Asbury, A. K., et al. Oculomotor palsy in diabetes mellitus: A clinicopathological study. *Brain* 93:955, 1970.

Burde, R. M., and Loewy, A. D. Central origin of oculomotor parasympathetic neurons in the monkey. *Brain Res.* 193:434, 1980.

Goldstein, J., and Cogan, D. Diabetic ophthalmoplegia with special reference to the pupil. *Arch. Ophthalmol.* 64:592, 1960.

Guy, J., et al. Superior division paresis of the oculomotor nerve. *Ophthalmology* 92:777, 1985.

Kissel, J. T., et al. Pupil-sparing oculomotor palsies with internal carotid–posterior communicating artery aneurysms. *Ann. Neurol.* 13:149, 1983.

Lepore, F. E., and Glaser, J. S. Misdirection revisited: A critical appraisal of acquired oculomotor nerve synkinesis. *Arch. Ophthalmol.* 98:2206, 1980.

O'Connor, P. S., Tredici, T. J., and Green, R. P. Pupil sparing third nerve palsies caused by aneurysm. *Am. J. Ophthalmol.* 95:395, 1983.

Rush, J. A., and Younge, B. R. Paralysis of cranial nerves III, IV, and VI: Cause and prognosis in 1,000 cases. *Arch. Ophthalmol.* 99:76, 1981.

Schatz, N. J., Savino, P. J., and Corbett, J. J. Primary aberrant oculomotor regeneration: A sign of intracavernous meningioma. *Arch. Neurol.* 34:29, 1977.

Sibony, P. A., Lessell, S., and Gittinger, J. W. Acquired oculomotor synkinesis. *Surv. Ophthalmol.* 28:382, 1984.

Trobe, J. D. Isolated pupil-sparing third nerve palsy. *Ophthalmology* 92:58, 1985.

Trobe, J. D., Glaser, J. S., and Post, J. D. Meningiomas, aneurysms of the cavernous sinus. *Arch. Ophthalmol.* 96:457, 1978.

25

Dorsal Midbrain Syndrome

An 18-year-old man went to a neurologist because of difficulty reading and headaches. These symptoms had become progressively worse over the previous 3 months. When his initial computed tomography (CT) scan was read as normal, he was referred with a tentative diagnosis of multiple sclerosis.

Neuro-Ophthalmic Examination

	OU
Visual acuity	20/20
Color plates correct	12 of 12
Pupils	7 mm and unreactive to light with a good near response
Motility	Absence of upgaze with nystagmus retractorius on attempted vertical saccades (up) (see p. 180)
Lids	Retracted
Orbits	Normal
Visual field	Normal
Fundi	Normal

Summary

An 18-year-old man manifested light-near pupillary dissociation, an inability to elevate either eye, and headaches.

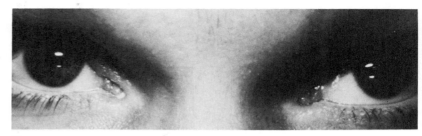

Upgaze

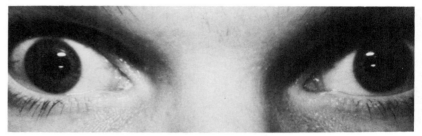

Primary position

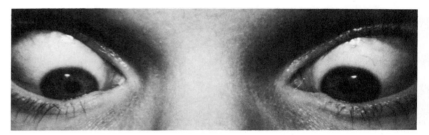

Downgaze

Differential Diagnosis

The findings of dilated pupils with light-near dissociation, upgaze paresis, nystagmus retractorius, and lid retraction define the dorsal midbrain syndrome (Parinaud's syndrome, sylvian aqueduct syndrome, pretectal syndrome, Koerber-Salus-Elschnig syndrome).

The first step in the differential diagnosis of this case is to recognize that the clinical findings are not orbital, that is, the patient does not have thyroid eye disease with restrictive upgaze bilaterally. The sluggish, dilated pupils and nystagmus are the tip-off that this is not a disease confined to the orbit. Brainstem syndromes as a result of a demyelinating process characteristically appear more acutely and tend not to worsen progressively as in this patient.

Clinical Diagnosis: Dorsal Midbrain Syndrome

Patients with a dorsal midbrain syndrome frequently develop a paresis of upgaze saccadic movements manifested clinically by oscillopsia when attempting to look up rapidly during reading, in work requiring scans of vision in the vertical plane, or in sports. As the syndrome progresses there are further complaints of oscillopsia and blurred vision as the nystagmus retractorius appears with attempts to maintain the primary position and on lateral saccades. This convergence-retraction movement of the eyes with any attempt to look up is thought to be caused by cofiring of muscles supplied by the third nerve nucleus as a result of either pressure or damage to the region of the posterior commissure. Because of the contiguous location of the third and fourth cranial nerve nuclei, these patients may also complain of vertical diplopia from skew deviation. Findings in the dorsal midbrain syndrome are:

1. Paresis of upgaze saccades
2. Disturbances of downward eye movements
3. Fixation instability
4. Skew deviation
5. Pupillary light-near dissociation (dilated sluggish pupils)
6. Lid retraction (Collier's sign)
7. Convergence-retraction nystagmus with attempted upgaze saccades
8. Papilledema (when the ventricular outflow has been obstructed)

Tumors, vascular lesions, and demyelinating disease involving the dorsal midbrain region can lead to this syndrome. A pinealoma, although classically described as the cause of Parinaud's syndrome, is found only in some cases. Atypical teratomas involving the region of the pineal gland are frequently a cause of the syndrome; these tumors are extremely radiosensitive and patients generally have good long-term survival with radiation therapy. Astrocytomas also may occur in this area.

Additional Testing

Before the advent of high-resolution CT scanning and magnetic resonance imaging (MRI), lesions of the posterior fossa were extremely difficult to image—a factor emphasizing the importance of good clinical localization. Now with the newer neuroimaging modalities the ability to localize the lesion clinically still remains important in aiming these powerful tools to avoid missed or delayed diagnosis.

Management and Course of the Case

Repeat CT scanning suggested the presence of a pineal region mass and hydrocephalus. The tumor was confirmed using metrizamide contrast with CT scanning, and with MRI (see p. 182). A biopsy of the lesion was performed and a shunt placed at the time of biopsy. Histologically, the tumor was found to be a dysgerminoma, one of the more common tumors to involve the pineal region. The tumor was treated with radiation therapy, and follow-up MRI has shown no recurrence during a 2-year period. The patient's symptoms of oscillopsia and difficulty in reading have persisted, but the headaches have ceased.

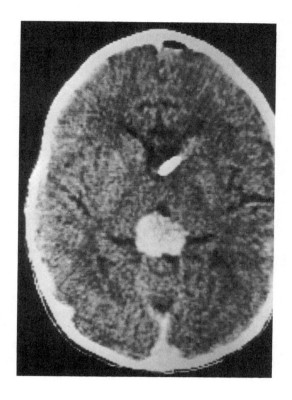

Bibliography

Baloh, R. W., Furman, J. M., and Yee, R. D. Dorsal midbrain syndrome: Clinical and oculographic findings. *Neurology* 35:54, 1985.

Case Records of the Massachusetts General Hospital (Case 25-1971). *N. Engl. J. Med.* 284:1427, 1971.

Case Records of the Massachusetts General Hospital (Case 35-1983). *N. Engl. J. Med.* 309:542, 1983.

Daroff, R. B., and Hoyt, W. F. Supranuclear Disorders of Ocular Control Systems in Man: Clinical, Anatomical, and Physiological Correlations—1969. In P. Bach-y-Rita, C. C. Collins, and J. E. Hyde (eds.), *The Control of Eye Movements.* New York: Academic, 1971. Pp. 175–235.

Daroff, R. B., and Troost, B. T. Supranuclear Disorders of Eye Movements. In J. S. Glaser (ed.), *Neuro-ophthalmology.* Hagerstown, Md.: Harper & Row, 1978. Pp. 201–218.

Gay, A. J., Brodkey, J., and Miller, J. E. Convergence retraction nystagmus: An electromyographic study. *Arch. Ophthalmol.* 70:456, 1963.

Miller, N. R. Topical Diagnosis of Neuropathic Ocular Motility Disorders. In *Walsh and Hoyt's Clinical Neuro-ophthalmology* (4th ed.). Baltimore: Williams & Wilkins, 1985. Vol. 2, pp. 716–719.

Parinaud, H. Paralysis of the movement of convergence of the eyes. *Brain* 9:330, 1886.

Pierrot-Deseilligny, C., et al. Parinaud's syndrome: Electro-oculographic and anatomical analyses of six vascular cases with deductions about vertical gaze organization in premotor structures. *Brain* 105:667, 1982.

Seybold, M. E., et al. Pupillary abnormalities associated with tumors of the pineal region. *Neurology* 21:232, 1971.

Smith, J. L., et al. Nystagmus retractorius. *Arch. Ophthalmol.* 62:864, 1959.

Thames, P. B., Trobe, J. D., and Ballinger, W. E. Upgaze paralysis caused by a lesion of the periaqueductal grey matter. *Arch. Neurol.* 41:437, 1984.

26

Skew Deviation

A 58-year-old man had the sudden onset of vertical diplopia, inability to walk, and headache. He had long-standing hypertension that had been untreated. He had also noted difficulty in swallowing his lunch shortly after the onset of his symptoms.

Neuro-Ophthalmic Examination

	OU
Visual acuity	20/20
Color plates correct	10 of 10
Pupils	Normal
Visual field	Normal
Fundi	Hypertensive changes
Motility	Coarse rotatory nystagmus on left gaze; fine horizontal jerk nystagmus on right gaze

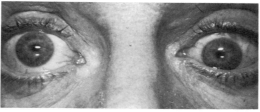

Primary position

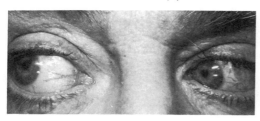

Right gaze

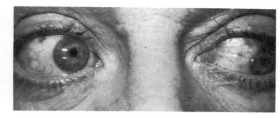

Left gaze

A neurologic examination showed left-sided ataxia with decreased palatal movement on the left.

Summary

A 58-year-old man with a long-standing history of untreated hypertension had the abrupt onset of vertical diplopia, difficulty swallowing, and ataxia.

Differential Diagnosis

The vertical diplopia and rotatory nystagmus, when coupled with hemiataxia and ipsilateral palatal dysfunction, precisely localize the lesion to the medullary region of the brainstem where oculomotor input fibers, tenth nerve nuclei, and cerebellar pathways converge. Although rotatory nystagmus and vertical diplopia (from otolith dysfunction) may occur in peripheral labyrinthine disturbances, the presence of concomitant long tract or cerebellar findings should always suggest a central lesion. When a vertical ocular separation is present on a brainstem basis and cannot be attributed to a specific extraocular muscle deficit, it is called *skew deviation.*

The abrupt onset of brainstem dysfunction and headache in a patient with hypertension should always alert the examiner to the possibility of a posterior fossa hemorrhage. However, ischemia by itself is frequently associated with occipital or retro-orbital head pain when involving the posterior circulation. When an infarction occurs in the distribution of the lateral medullary plate region, it is generally a result of vertebral artery atherosclerosis.

Clinical Diagnosis: Brainstem Vascular Insult Producing Skew Deviation

Skew deviation is a vertical misalignment of the eyes that cannot be explained on the basis of extraocular muscle dysfunction or an ocular motor nerve palsy. Unlike a fourth nerve paresis, skew deviation does not generally have an associated cyclodeviation or torsional diplopia. The basis for the misalignment is an abnormality of the prenuclear inputs in the brainstem. Individuals with true skew deviation will almost always have other brainstem findings on careful neurologic examination.

Skew can be either concomitant (constant in all positions of gaze) or nonconcomitant (e.g., right hypertropia on right gaze, left hypertropia on left gaze). Not infrequently, a unilateral internuclear ophthalmoplegia is seen on the side of the hypertropia. The pathophysiology of the skew deviation is thought to be dysfunction of the otolith inputs in the medulla. Although skew deviations have been seen with peripheral lesions involving the otolith output, the presence of other focal brainstem findings in this patient clearly localizes the lesion to the region of the medulla. The lower eye in the skew deviation will more commonly be on the side of the brainstem lesion, as noted in this patient with the left eye lower and the ataxia and palatal dysfunction present ipsilaterally.

Additional Testing and Management

Once a skew deviation has been identified, the appropriate neuroimaging techniques should be employed to outline the type of brainstem pathology present. Such testing is particularly urgent in the patient with a posterior fossa hemorrhage involving the cerebellum, in which case surgical decompression may be lifesaving. For the ischemic insult the treatment is primarily supportive, although with serious swelling surgical decompression may be indicated to prevent herniation.

Management and Course of the Case

A computed tomography scan was obtained that demonstrated an incidental anterior communicating artery aneurysm. No hemorrhage was seen in the region of the brainstem. Four-vessel intraarterial digital subtraction angiography confirmed the presence of the aneurysm along with a completely occluded left vertebral artery. Over a period of 3 months the patient's neurologic deficits resolved entirely. During the surgical attempt to clip his aneurysm he had a cardiac arrest and died. At autopsy the vertebral artery occlusion was confirmed, with a well-demarcated infarct involving the lateral medullary plate region.

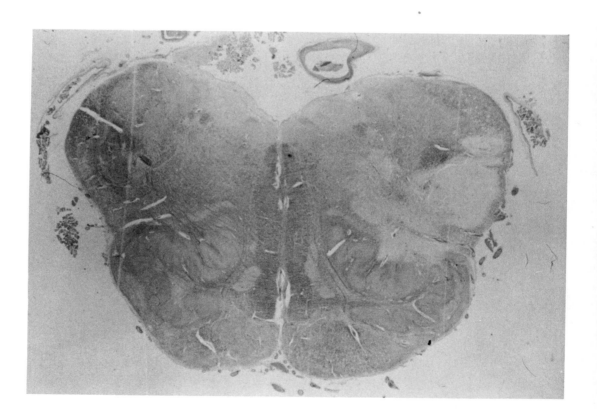

Bibliography

Keane, J. R. Ocular skew deviation. *Arch. Neurol.* 32:185, 1975.

Mitchell, J. M., Smith, J. L., and Quencer, R. M. Periodic alternating skew deviation. *J. Clin. Neuro Ophthalmol.* 1:5, 1981.

Nashold, B. S., and Seaber, J. H. Defects of ocular motility after stereotactic midbrain lesions in man. *Arch. Ophthalmol.* 88:245, 1972.

Smith, J. L., David, N. J., and Klintworth, G. Skew deviation. *Neurology* 14:96, 1964.

Trobe, J. D. Cyclodeviation in acquired vertical strabismus. *Arch. Ophthalmol.* 102:717, 1984.

27

Sixth Nerve Palsy

A 65-year-old man noted the abrupt onset of horizontal diplopia and dysequilibrium shortly after awakening. A mild left retro-orbital aching pain had awakened him earlier that morning. His medical history was otherwise unremarkable; he had not seen a physician for more than 20 years.

Neuro-Ophthalmic Examination

	OU
Visual acuity	20/20
Color plates correct	12 of 12
Pupils	4 mm
Visual field	Normal
Fundi	Hypertensive vascular changes

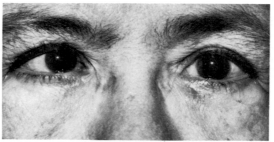

Primary position

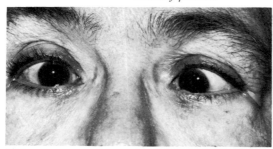

Right gaze

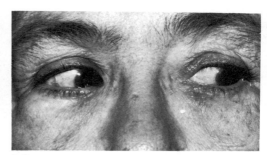

Left gaze

Results of a neurologic examination were normal except for a blood pressure of 160/98. Vertical gaze was normal.

Summary

A 65-year-old man had the abrupt onset of an abduction deficit associated with mild retro-orbital pain.

Differential Diagnosis

The initial step in the assessment of an abduction deficit is to determine whether the disorder is one of muscle, neuromuscular junction, nerve, or brainstem. Too often the diagnosis of a sixth nerve paresis is made without consideration of other causes.

Forced duction tests are required to determine if the medial rectus is entrapped or tethered in the orbit. Although ocular myasthenia may occasionally present as an isolated abduction deficit, other ocular findings are usually present and serve as a clue to the presence of this disease. A Tensilon test should be undertaken if there is any suggestion by history or exam of myasthenia gravis.

Other conditions that may mimic a sixth nerve paresis are listed with their differentiating features in Table 27-1.

In this patient a forced duction test and a Tensilon test had normal results; thus ocular myasthenia and a restrictive process were unlikely. The retraction seen with Duane's syndrome was not observed on motility testing, and the absence of pupillary constriction on attempted left gaze indicated the absence of convergence spasm. It was only by a process of elimination that the patient was suspected of having a sixth nerve paresis.

Table 27-1. Differential diagnosis of an abduction deficit

Entity	Differentiating features
I. Muscle	
A. Myopathy	Other ocular or facial muscle involvement
B. Restrictive disease	Systemic signs, neuroimaging evidence of
1. Graves' ophthalmopathy	muscle enlargement or fracture, positive
2. Myositis	forced duction results
3. Blowout fracture	
II. Neuromuscular junction: myasthenia gravis	Tensilon test results, other ocular or facial muscle involvement
III. Nuclear: Duane's retraction syndrome	Characteristic retraction of the globe on adduction, lid closure on adduction
IV. Other causes	
A. Convergence spasm	Pupillary constriction with attempted lateral gaze
B. Congenital esotropia	Concomitance of the deviation

Clinical Diagnosis: Sixth Nerve Paresis

The abducens nerves arise from motor cells that lie on the floor of the fourth ventricle adjacent to the fascicles of the facial nerve that arc posterolaterally as the facial colliculi. The lateral rectus innervation originates from the central aspect of this group of cells; the surrounding cells in the nuclei make up the paraabducens nuclei, centers for horizontal conjugate gaze.

The abducens fascicles course ventrally through the pontine tegmentum to exit ventromedially at the pontomedullary junction. After exiting the brainstem they turn rostrally over the tips of the petrous pyramids (in Dorello's canal) to enter the cavernous sinuses adjacent to the carotid arteries. From the cavernous sinus the sixth nerve then enters the orbits through the superior orbital fissures in proximity to the third, fourth, and sympathetic nerve inputs.

Once it has been established that an abduction deficit is secondary to a sixth nerve paresis, then a careful neurologic examination is necessary to look for other evidence of cranial nerve dysfunction or increased intracranial pressure. The course of the sixth cranial nerve takes it in proximity to many brain, bony, and sinus structures. Lesions affecting the abducens nucleus or fascicle exiting the brainstem usually involve ipsilateral facial nerve function and may produce a conjugate gaze paresis toward the side of the lesion (Foville's syndrome) from involvement of the contiguous facial nerve fascicle or the paraabducens nucleus. Lesions involving the sixth nerve in its course through the cavernous sinus may also affect the third or fourth cranial nerves or involve the autonomic supply to the eye, giving rise to a characteristic cavernous sinus syndrome. The sixth nerve is vulnerable to changes in intracranial pressure, possibly through a traction phenomenon as it enters Dorello's canal. A sixth nerve paresis in patients with elevated intracranial pressure from any cause, after lumbar puncture, or after myelography may therefore represent a *false localizing sign*.

Paresis of the sixth cranial nerve is the most frequently reported ocular motor paresis and, when an isolated finding in a patient over the age of 40, usually represents an infarction of the nerve trunk from the small vessel disease of diabetes or hypertension. Bilateral sixth nerve palsies, however, are almost never from vascular disease and should be evaluated as outlined below.

In children, postviral syndromes, trauma, and neoplastic disease account for the majority of sixth nerve paresis. The most common tumor in the younger age groups is the brainstem glioma.

Table 27-2. Management of isolated sixth nerve paresis

Age group	Unilateral	Bilateral
Children	Follow only	Follow or perform MRI
Young adult	Perform CT or MRI, vasculitis workup, VDRL test, and LP	Same as for unilateral
Older adult	Obtain BP, fasting blood sugar measurements	Perform CT or MRI; if normal, LP

Key: MRI = magnetic resonance imaging; CT = computed tomography; LP = lumbar puncture; BP = blood pressure.

Additional Testing and Management

The management of an isolated, nontraumatic, unilateral sixth nerve paresis depends on the age of the patient, as reviewed in Table 27-2.

In the pediatric age group, close clinical follow-up without extensive investigation is advised. In those over the age of 50, close attention to the blood pressure, screening for diabetes, and close clinical follow-up will circumvent costly neurodiagnostic procedures with much the same in the way of diagnostic yield. In the young adult the management becomes a bit more controversial. It is our policy to perform magnetic resonance imaging (MRI) to look for a basal skull lesion if blood testing reveals no systemic cause for the mononeuropathy. In adults of any age, neuroimaging should be obtained when a bilateral sixth nerve paresis is seen unassociated with pseudotumor cerebri, or after lumbar puncture or myelography.

In any age group, progression of the sixth nerve paresis, development of additional signs, or the lack of any improvement within 3 months mandates a neuroradiologic workup.

The treatment of the diplopia produced by a sixth nerve paresis consists of either patching one eye or using Fresnel prisms if the deficit is expected to be of long duration. Extraocular muscle surgery should not be considered unless a deviation has been stable for at least 6 months. The role of botulinum injections is controversial.

Management and Course of the Case

The patient was treated with an eye patch and analgesics. The fasting blood sugar level was 87 mg/dl, and his blood pressure remained high on numerous examinations. He was treated with a beta blocker for his hypertension. No neuroimaging studies were performed. The abduction deficit resolved completely over a 6-week period.

Limited Abduction from Graves' Ophthalmopathy

An 82-year-old woman had worsening diplopia over a period of several months. The diplopia was described as horizontal, initially intermittent, and recently associated with a "pulling" sensation with attempted extremes of gaze.

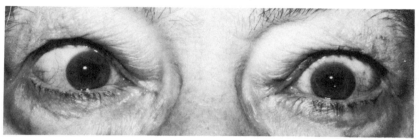

Primary position

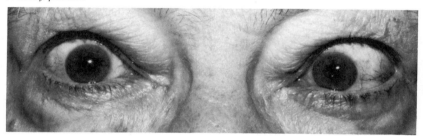

Right gaze

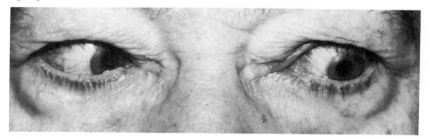

Left gaze

On examination limitation of upgaze and abduction was noted, with positive results on forced duction testing suggesting restrictive ophthalmopathy. Although no proptosis was noted there was lid retraction. Visual acuity was 20/20 in each eye, and the funduscopic appearance was unremarkable. An orbital computed tomography (CT) scan showed bilateral extraocular muscle enlargement.

This patient has an abduction deficit from the restrictive ophthalmopathy of dysthyroid orbitopathy. This diagnosis should have been apparent from the results of the forced duction testing and the lid retraction present on examination. (See Chapter 22 for a discussion of Graves' ophthalmopathy.)

Duane's Retraction Syndrome

A 23-year-old woman was referred because of headaches and what had been diagnosed as a sixth nerve paresis. Multiple diagnostic tests had failed to reveal any abnormalities. She stated that she had always had "weak eyes" but denied symptoms of diplopia. Her medical history was otherwise unremarkable.

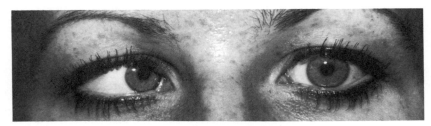

Left gaze

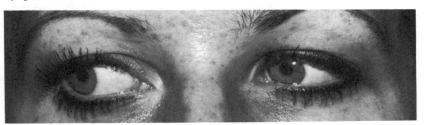

Right gaze

A left abduction deficit with upward deviation of each adducting eye was seen. Globe retraction and palpebral fissure narrowing were noted on attempted adduction bilaterally. Forced duction testing results were equivocal for a restrictive component to the abduction deficit.

This patient has congenital Duane's retraction syndrome. This syndrome is classified into three types. Type 1, the most commonly seen, involves limitation of abduction with full adduction. Type 2 is characterized by intact abduction with incomplete adduction. Abduction and adduction are both limited in type 3. All types are characterized by palpebral fissure narrowing with attempted adduction. The abducens nucleus fails to develop normally in Duane's retraction syndrome, the result of which is a redirection of the innervation of the extraocular muscles.

In Duane's retraction syndrome, the eyes are often straight despite an inability to abduct beyond the midline. This finding is the tip-off to the diagnosis since with a complete sixth nerve palsy there will always be esotropia in the primary position.

Convergence Spasm

An 18-year-old woman was seen with complaints of eye pain and diplopia. She had undergone a CT scan, MRI, an electroencephalogram, a Tensilon test, and lumbar puncture—all of which had normal results. On examination she demonstrated abduction deficits more pronounced on right than left gaze. With attempts at lateral gaze the pupils promptly constricted. Saccadic movements elicited with the optokinetic tape were carried out normally, as were her eye movements when looking about the clinic waiting room.

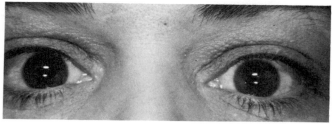

Primary position

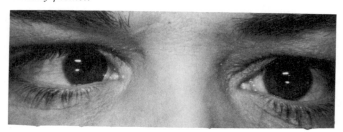

Left gaze

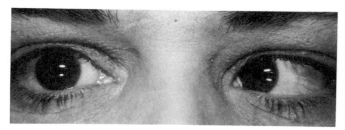

Right gaze

This patient is clearly using convergence as a mechanism to prevent her abducting eye from carrying out a full excursion. The prompt constriction of the pupils on lateral gaze confirms the presence of convergence spasm (spasm of the near reflex).

An abduction deficit is too often an unwarranted invitation to extensive neuroradiologic evaluation. Panic is created in the best of clinicians when bilateral abduction deficits are seen. Emergency and extensive investigations, such as occurred with this patient, are promptly arranged. Unfortunately, a unilateral or, more commonly, a bilateral abduction deficit can be easily mimicked by anyone with a strong degree of convergence and with the tenacity to sustain this convergence through repeated examinations.

Convergence spasm, or spasm of the near reflex, is characterized by intermittent and usually painful convergence, accommodation, and miosis. Although it has been reported with underlying disorders of the vestibular system or brainstem, it is almost invariably attributed to hysteria. In our experience, the majority of these patients have a history of minor head trauma followed by major legal involvement.

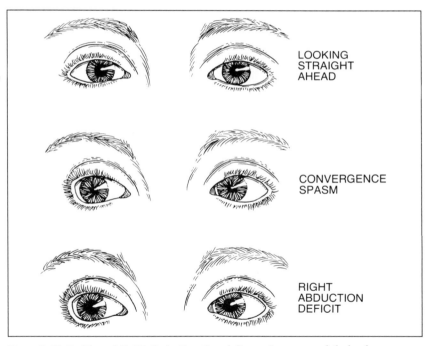

LOOKING STRAIGHT AHEAD

CONVERGENCE SPASM

RIGHT ABDUCTION DEFICIT

From C. H. Smith and R. W. Beck. Functional disease in neuro-ophthalmology. Neurol. Clin. 1:955, 1983. Reprinted with permission from W. B. Saunders Co.

The esotropia of convergence spasm may be asymmetric in extent and variable in degree when measured by prisms. Full abduction may be noted on saccade or oculocephalic testing. Patching or cycloplegic drops may enable the examiner to frustrate the patient's attempts at maintaining the convergence spasm.

Bibliography

Bajandas, F. J. The Six Syndromes of the Sixth Nerve. In J. L. Smith (ed.), *Neuro-ophthalmology Update.* New York: Masson, 1977. Pp. 49–67.

Harley, R. Paralytic strabismus in children: Etiologic incidence and management of the third, fourth and sixth nerve palsies. *Ophthalmology* 87:24, 1980.

Isenberg, S., and Urist, M. J. Clinical observations in 101 consecutive patients with Duane's retraction syndrome. *Am. J. Ophthalmol.* 84:419, 1977.

Keane, J. R. Bilateral sixth nerve palsy. *Arch. Neurol.* 33:681, 1976.

Kline, L. B. *Neuro-ophthalmology Review Manual* (2nd ed.). Thorofare, N.J.: Slack, 1987.

Miller, N. R., et al. Unilateral Duane's retraction syndrome (type 1). *Arch. Ophthalmol.* 100:1468, 1982.

Rush, J. A., and Younge, B. R. Paralysis of cranial nerves III, IV, and VI: Cause and prognosis in 1,000 cases. *Arch. Ophthalmol.* 99:76, 1981.

Savino, P. J., et al. Chronic sixth nerve palsies. *Arch. Ophthalmol.* 100:1442, 1982.

Smith, C. H., Beck, R. W., and Mills, R. P. Functional disease in neuro-ophthalmology. *Neurol. Clin.* 1:955, 1983.

28

Internuclear Ophthalmoplegia

A 25-year-old woman noted the abrupt onset of horizontal diplopia associated with unsteadiness and oscillopsia. Two years previously she had experienced an episode of dysequilibrium and right arm numbness lasting 2 weeks. Her only other complaint was that of urinary urgency, which had been treated on multiple occasions with antibiotics without success.

Neuro-Ophthalmic Examination

	OU
Visual acuity	20/20
Color plates correct	12 of 12
Pupils	Normal
Fundi	Normal
Motility	Coarse vertical nystagmus on upgaze in both eyes, horizontal nystagmus in abduction of right eye

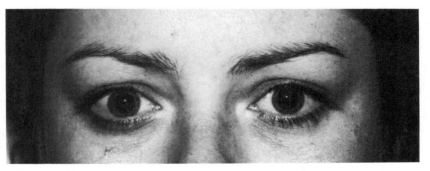

Primary position

Upgaze and downgaze were normal.

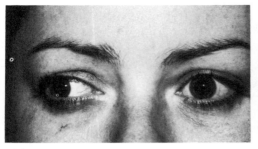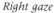
Right gaze

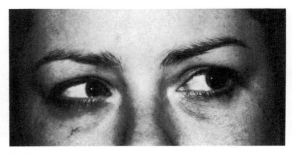
Left gaze

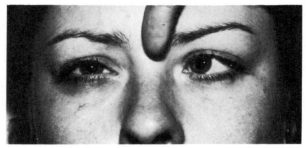
Convergence

Neurologic examination showed mild dysmetria in the arms with brisk reflexes and positive Babinski signs bilaterally.

Summary

A young woman had an adduction deficit on the left associated with vertical nystagmus, cerebellar findings, and positive Babinski responses.

Differential Diagnosis

Adduction deficits can be caused by disorders of the muscle, neuromuscular junction, or brainstem. Isolated lateral rectus restriction leading to an ipsilateral adduction deficit is rarely seen without other evidence of orbital disease. A third nerve paresis manifesting solely as a medial rectus deficit is rarely seen. The major differential of an isolated adduction deficit is between internuclear ophthalmoplegia (INO) and myasthenia gravis (Table 28-1).

Table 28-1. Causes of adduction deficits

Disorder of	Cause
Muscle	Restrictive syndromes such as dysthyroid orbitopathy
Neuromuscular junction	Ocular myasthenia
Nerve	Branch third nerve paresis (ischemic, inflammatory, compressive)
Brainstem	Internuclear ophthalmoplegia

The presence of slowed saccades in a paretic adducting eye suggests internuclear ophthalmoplegia and is contrasted with the normal saccade with a quick stop encountered in the tethered eye in restrictive ophthalmopathy and the initial rapid saccade in myasthenia gravis. The absence of ptosis, other evidence of ophthalmoplegia, or myasthenic features on general neurologic examination points away from a disorder of the neuromuscular junction.

This patient clearly has other "signatures" of brainstem dysfunction—cerebellar and pyramidal tract signs and symptoms. The presence of an adduction deficit without other evidence of third nerve nuclear involvement suggests the involvement of the brainstem internuclear pathways between the paraabducens and third nerve nuclei in the region of the medial longitudinal fasciculus (MLF) leading to INO.

Clinical Diagnosis: Internuclear Ophthalmoplegia

Horizontal gaze is mediated by neurons in the region of the paraabducens nuclear group in the pons. Interneurons in the paraabducens area project from the abducens nuclei to the contralateral third nerve nuclei. These projections travel in the medial longitudinal fasciculus, providing excitatory and inhibitory input to the oculomotor muscles. In this manner, excitation of a paraabducens region by supranuclear (cortical) input leads to ipsilateral sixth and contralateral third nerve excitation and inhibition of the ipsilateral third and contralateral sixth nerves. Stimulation of the right paraabducens nucleus produces gaze in each eye to the right, and stimulation of the left nucleus produces gaze to the left.

Complete lesions of the MLF lead to loss of adduction with preserved abduction. Convergence may be normal or impaired. The eyes are often straight in the primary position even when there is a complete inability to adduct.

Partial lesions of the MLF may lead to a lag of the adducting eye when compared with the abducting eye when saccadic movements are carried out. This type of "subclinical" internuclear ophthalmoplegia is best seen clinically by the use of the optokinetic tape, observing the synchrony of the two eyes during the quick phases of refixation. In a subclinical INO, the adducting eye on the side of the brainstem lesion will lag in comparison to the abducting eye during the quick component of optokinetic nystagmus. When observed closely, many seemingly unilateral INOs are actually bilateral but asymmetric in the degree of involvement of the two sides.

In INO, nystagmus is seen in the abducting eye, possibly as a result of altered inhibitory input to the lateral rectus muscle. (This abducting-eye nystagmus can also be seen in the pseudo-INO of ocular myasthenia.) In addition, vertical nystagmus is frequently seen in unilateral or bilateral INO.

When truly unilateral, INO suggests vascular disease, particularly when it has an abrupt onset in the older population. Bilateral INO is most frequently seen in demyelinating disease (multiple sclerosis [MS]).

Although great emphasis has been placed on classifying INOs into anterior and posterior varieties, accompanying signs usually localize the lesion independently of the presence of the INO.

In this patient the presence of brainstem findings with a history of transient neurologic symptoms suggests the diagnosis of demyelinating disease (MS), which, by definition, consists of lesions in the nervous system "separated in time and space."

INO is rarely the sole presenting feature of multiple sclerosis. As seen with this patient, other signs are usually found on neurologic examination, or clues are given in the patient's history to suggest the diagnosis. For example, symptoms of urinary urgency or frequency are commonly elicited, which suggest lesions involving the descending pathways subserving bladder control. As indicated in Chapter 1, the history is a very important aspect of the neuro-ophthalmic evaluation.

Additional Testing

The neuroimaging modality of choice for the evaluation of the posterior fossa is magnetic resonance imaging (MRI). Not only does MRI show the brainstem better than computed tomography (CT), MRI may also provide additional evidence of multiple sclerosis lesions in the periventricular region of the cortex without additional charge to the patient. However, even with MRI evidence of white matter lesions typical of those seen in multiple sclerosis, cerebrospinal fluid (CSF) examination may be necessary to rule out treatable infectious causes. Opportunistic infections in younger patients with acquired immune deficiency states may have MRI evidence of white matter lesions similar to those seen in MS.

Treatment

The diplopia seen in INO is usually transient when the underlying pathology is a demyelinating process. In the symptomatic patient an eye patch is all that is required.

There is no known treatment for multiple sclerosis. Corticosteroids, chemotherapy, hyperbaric oxygen, plasmapheresis, and a variety of other therapies have been tried, but no evidence has been presented that confirms their effectiveness in the long-term management of the disease. Regular exercise, good nutrition, and good patient understanding of the disease are paramount in maintaining a good quality of life with multiple sclerosis.

Management and Course of the Case

CT scan showed multiple low-density lesions involving the white matter of both hemispheres. MRI confirmed the presence of water-density lesions scattered extensively throughout the cortical white matter. CSF analysis showed a protein of 45 mg/dl, elevated titers of myelin basic protein, and the presence of oligoclonal banding. These findings all strongly suggested the diagnosis of multiple sclerosis.

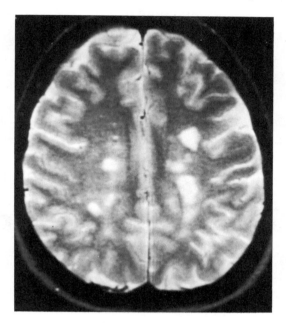

The patient was given no treatment, and her findings resolved gradually over the subsequent 1 month. Six months later she developed left optic neuritis and myelopathy, leaving her wheelchair bound.

Bilateral Internuclear Ophthalmoplegia

A 33-year-old woman abruptly noticed horizontal diplopia while driving. She had been diagnosed as having optic neuritis on two occasions in the previous 2 years. On review of systems, she complained of urinary frequency and urgency but denied any other neurologic symptoms.

On examination she was orthophoric in the primary position with bilateral adduction defects and abducting nystagmus. Vertical gaze was normal. Her neurologic examination disclosed diffuse hyperreflexia and bilateral Babinski responses. Abdominal reflexes were absent. MRI, on a T_2 weighted study, demonstrated multiple water-density lesions in the white matter of both hemispheres, consistent with the diagnosis of a demyelinating disease.

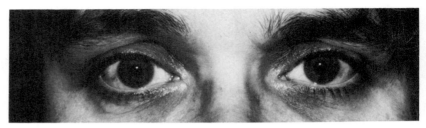

Primary position

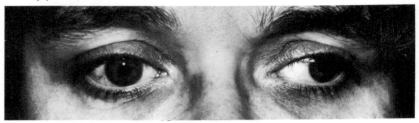

Left gaze

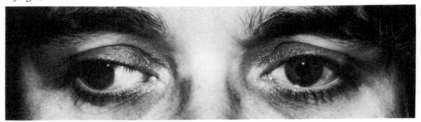

Right gaze

In this setting the presence of bilateral INO is virtually pathognomonic for a demyelinating process, so much so that MRI becomes a costly, redundant tool in the management of the disease. With a clear history of central nervous system lesions separated in space and time, the presence of bilateral INO should do no more than alert the examiner to the presence of active demyelinating disease.

Walleyed Bilateral Internuclear Ophthalmoplegia

A 58-year-old woman noted the abrupt onset of diplopia and dysequilibrium while driving. Her medical history included untreated hypertension, which she claimed to have had for more than 30 years.

On examination her eyes were divergent with a left hypertropia of 12 diopters. She demonstrated a bilateral adduction deficit with absence of convergence.

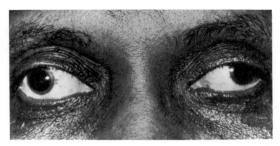

Primary position

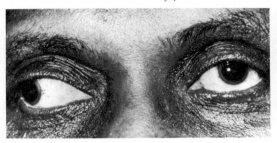

Right gaze

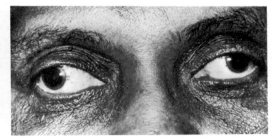

Left gaze

This case is an example of walleyed bilateral internuclear ophthalmoplegia (WEBINO). Lesions causing a WEBINO syndrome are present in the rostral MLF of the mesencephalon, are bilateral, and are characterized by an absence of convergence with exotropic gaze. In this patient the underlying pathophysiology was a small vessel infarct secondary to long-standing hypertension. Since the vascular disease involved the posterior circulation, no arteriographic studies were obtained. The patient's hypertension was treated, with gradual clearing of her deficits.

Adduction Deficit from Myasthenia Gravis

A 45-year-old man had had horizontal diplopia for 2 months. He noted it especially in the afternoons while driving a mail truck. He had noted fatigue on chewing and some difficulty in walking up a flight of stairs during the foregoing year. His medical history was otherwise unremarkable, except for hypothyroidism treated with replacement medication.

On examination he had bilateral adduction deficits with hypertropia and nystagmus of the abducting eye to either side. Minimal ptosis was noted. Immediately after the injection of a 2-mg test dose of Tensilon there was complete clearing of the ocular findings.

As mentioned previously, myasthenia gravis may mimic any ocular motor disorder. In this case, ocular myasthenia produced a pseudo-INO. The tip-off to the neuromuscular nature of the ocular motor deficit was twofold: first, the end-of-day fatigability, and second, the ptosis and prominent vertical deviation of the abducting eyes, which are unusual for INO. While there may be a skew deviation in INO it generally is not of large amplitude. Ptosis is rarely seen in INO. When in doubt, test with Tensilon!

Bibliography

Crane, T. B., et al. Analysis of characteristic eye movement abnormalities in internuclear ophthalmoplegia. *Arch. Ophthalmol.* 101:206, 1983.

Daroff, R. B., and Hoyt, W. F. Supranuclear Disorders of Ocular Control Systems in Man: Clinical, Anatomical, and Physiological Correlations—1969. In P. Bach-y-Rita, C. C. Collins, and J. E. Hyde (eds.), *The Control of Eye Movements.* New York: Academic, 1971. Pp. 175–235.

Dell'Osso, L. F., Robinson, D. A., and Daroff, R. B. Optokinetic asymmetry in internuclear ophthalmoplegia. *Arch. Neurol.* 31:138, 1974.

Glaser, J. S. Myasthenic pseudo-internuclear ophthalmoplegia. *Arch. Ophthalmol.* 75:363, 1966.

Gonyea, E. F. Bilateral internuclear ophthalmoplegia. *Arch. Neurol.* 31:168, 1974.

Kommerell, G. Internuclear ophthalmoplegia of abduction: Isolated impairment of phasic ocular motor activity in supranuclear lesions. *Arch. Ophthalmol.* 93:531, 1975.

Kommerell, G. Unilateral internuclear ophthalmoplegia: The lack of inhibitory involvement in medial rectus muscle activity. *Invest. Ophthalmol. Vis. Sci.* 21:592, 1981.

Muri, R. M., and Meienberg, O. The clinical spectrum of internuclear ophthalmoplegia in multiple sclerosis. *Arch. Neurol.* 42:851, 1985.

Wall, M., and Wray, S. H. The one-and-a-half syndrome—A unilateral disorder of the pontine tegmentum: A study of 20 cases and review of the literature. *Neurology* 33:971, 1983.

29

Fisher's Syndrome

A 13-year-old girl noted difficulty chewing food and horizontal diplopia that came on gradually over a period of 1 week. She had had a viral syndrome characterized by cough, sore throat, and malaise 2 weeks earlier. No history was given of ingested canned food or family members with a similar illness.

Neuro-Ophthalmic Examination

	OD	OS
Visual acuity	20/20	20/20
Color plates correct	12 of 12	12 of 12
Pupils	6 mm (sluggish)	6 mm (sluggish)
Optic disks	Normal	Normal
Visual field	Normal	Normal

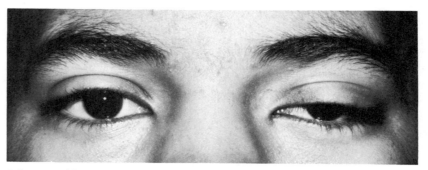

Primary position

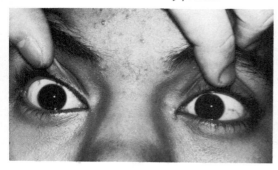

Right gaze

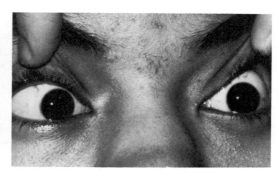

Left gaze

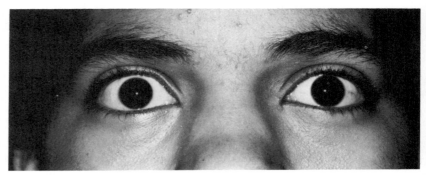

Upgaze

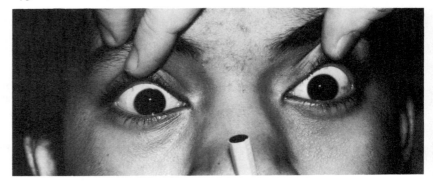

Downgaze

A general neurologic examination revealed facial diplegia, mild ataxia, and absent deep tendon reflexes.

Summary
A 13-year-old girl developed ophthalmoplegia, facial diplegia, and ataxia after a viral syndrome.

Differential Diagnosis
The differential diagnosis of subacute-onset ophthalmoparesis should include the same considerations of muscle, neuromuscular junction, nerve fascicle, and brainstem disease as outlined in Chapters 27 and 28. The presence of bilateral ophthalmoparesis and dilated poorly reactive pupils suggests a polyneuropathy involving the cranial nerves and rules out myasthenia or a myopathic process. The concomitant presence of cerebellar findings and areflexia indicate a widespread nervous system disorder.

Disorders of multiple cranial nerves involving the pupils but sparing other aspects of the central and peripheral nervous system include invasive skull base tumors, pituitary apoplexy, botulism, and the Guillain-Barré syndrome. The absence of pain and rapidity of onset in this case are against the diagnosis of an infiltrating lesion involving both cavernous sinuses. Ophthalmoparesis associated with dilated, sluggishly reactive pupils, particularly in association with a dry mouth and swallowing difficulties, should always alert the clinician to the possibility of botulism. Since the treatment of botulism should be initiated early with supportive ventilatory care, this diagnosis should be considered early with the appropriate cultures and animal inoculations. In this patient there is no historic evidence of exposure that would suggest botulism as a diagnosis.

The constellation of findings in this patient is most suggestive of a diagnosis of Fisher's syndrome.

Clinical Diagnosis: Fisher's Syndrome

The Guillain-Barré syndrome may present with ophthalmoparesis, ataxia, and areflexia—without weakness or respiratory symptoms. First described by Fisher in 1956, this variant of the Guillain-Barré syndrome (Fisher's syndrome) may include facial diplegia along with the ophthalmoparesis. The degree of ophthalmoparesis is variable; it may resemble a vertical or horizontal gaze paresis or internuclear ophthalmoplegia. Pupils may be normal or dilated, and when pharmacologic testing is performed, evidence of denervation hypersensitivity may be present, suggesting postganglionic or parasympathetic involvement.

Patients should be closely monitored for progression to include respiratory involvement in Fisher's syndrome, although in our experience this is an unusual occurrence. The pathophysiology in Fisher's variant of the Guillain-Barré syndrome is presumed to be a postviral lymphocyte-mediated demyelination of the nerve roots, although the pattern of ocular muscle involvement often suggests a central process. Whether or not there is involvement of the brainstem is a matter that has been hotly debated in the literature; as with any generalized insult involving the immunologic system, a combination of central and peripheral nervous system involvement is quite possible.

Additional Testing

The diagnosis of Fisher's syndrome is based on the clinical findings. Results of computed tomography (CT) or magnetic resonance imaging of the posterior fossa are normal. Cerebrospinal fluid (CSF) protein is often, but not always, elevated. A high protein count with little cellular reaction in the CSF (*albuminocytologic dissociation*) can also be seen in the presence of diphtheritic or diabetic polyneuropathy and should not, by itself, be taken as diagnostic of a Guillain-Barré variant.

Electrophysiologic testing of muscle and nerve may yield normal results or show evidence of denervation in Fisher's syndrome of long duration. These tests are not often helpful in acutely diagnosing the disease, but they may be an indicator of extent of axonal injury and, therefore, a predictor of chronicity.

Management

The treatment of Fisher's syndrome is supportive only and can usually be carried out on an outpatient basis, particularly if the patient's symptoms have stabilized. It must be remembered, however, that until the illness has stabilized there is a potential for respiratory distress. It is our policy to hospitalize any patient with Fisher's syndrome who is demonstrating progression in weakness or has any reduction in predicted pulmonary parameters. These patients may demonstrate other evidence of autonomic nervous system involvement: decreased bowel motility, disorders of sweating or temperature regulation, and cardiac arrythmias.

The use of corticosteroids and plasmapheresis in Fisher's syndrome is unwarranted in our opinion.

The typical course of Fisher's syndrome is complete resolution over a period of 4 to 12 weeks.

Management and Course of the Case

A lumbar puncture was obtained demonstrating a CSF protein level of 80 mg/dl without cellular response. Measurement of nerve conduction velocities, performed 3 weeks after the onset of symptoms, suggested a demyelinating polyneuropathy consistent with the diagnosis of Fisher's syndrome. The patient was not treated, and her symptoms cleared entirely over a 3-month period.

Chronic Progressive External Ophthalmoplegia

A 48-year-old woman was found by her optometrist to have difficulty moving her eyes. She denied a history of diplopia but did state that she had noted increasing difficulty with reading. Her family history was negative for neuromuscular illness. She had had a skin melanoma removed 5 years previously.

On examination she had minimal weakness in orbicularis oculi function with bilateral ptosis and a generalized ophthalmoparesis. General neurologic examination showed mild gait instability. No retinopathy was noted, and a cardiac examination had normal results.

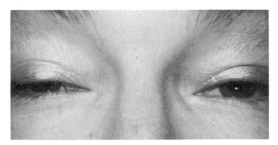

Primary position

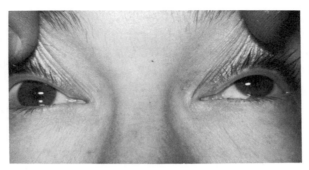

Upgaze

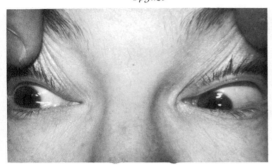

Right gaze

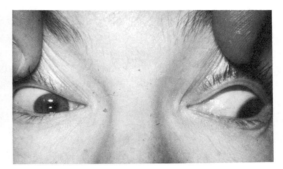

Left gaze

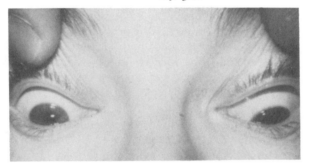

Downgaze

Causes of progressive limitation of ocular motility include:

1. Endocrine ophthalmoparesis
2. Myasthenia gravis
3. Oculopharyngeal dystrophy
4. Kearns-Sayre syndrome
5. Myotubular myopathy
6. Myotonic dystrophy
7. Bassen-Kornzweig syndrome

Although the term chronic progressive external ophthalmoplegia (CPEO) is often used to encompass all the slowly progressive external ophthalmoplegias, there is a subcategory—the distinct entity of the Kearns-Sayre syndrome—defined by the triad of ophthalmoplegia, pigmentary degeneration of the retina, and heart block. The retinal findings are an atypical retinitis pigmentosa (no true bone spicule formation), and the cardiopathy may not be present in the early years of the disease. The pathophysiology of this disease appears to be a defect of mitochondria, and the genetic transmission, while at times appearing to be classic autosomal dominant, may at other times be sporadic in appearance. Maternal mitochondrial cytoplasmic inheritance is felt to be a mechanism of transmission in the disease.

The patient's course was one of progressive ophthalmoplegia with the appearance of moderate difficulty swallowing and proximal muscle weakness. Muscle biopsy showed excessive ragged red fibers with trichrome staining methods, findings seen in Kearns-Sayre syndrome.

The histologic findings of mitochondrial myopathy in this patient without the typical clinical findings of Kearns-Sayre syndrome serve to point out that a pure form of the disease is the exception.

Oculopharyngeal Muscular Dystrophy

A 39-year-old French Canadian man presented with ptosis and difficulty reading. He complained of progressive difficulty in swallowing over a 1-year period. His father had had similar symptoms in his thirties and had died suddenly from aspirating a chunk of meat.

Neuro-ophthalmic examination showed ptosis and almost a complete external ophthalmoplegia with good pupillary responses. Temporal wasting and neck flexor weakness were present, as well as decreased motility on esophageal barium swallow. Forced duction and Tensilon testing had negative results.

This patient manifests the clinical findings seen in oculopharyngeal muscular dystrophy. This is a primary disorder of muscle that first presents in the forties, frequently in families of French Canadian heritage, and with an autosomal dominant inheritance pattern. These patients may have dysphagia for years before the appearance of the ptosis and ophthalmoparesis. The ptosis is typically symmetric, although several of our patients have initially had unilateral ptosis; the diagnosis is never in question with a family history and concomitant neurologic findings. Muscle biopsy in these patients shows a marked reduction in muscle fibers with vacuolation and nuclear inclusions. There is no specific treatment, although cricopharyngeal myotomy has helped some patients with swallowing, thus improving their quality of life.

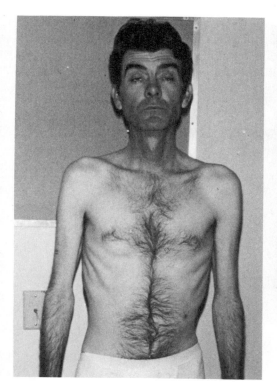 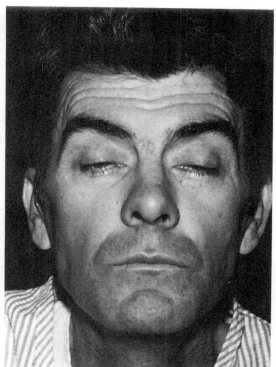

A 36-year-old man had diplopia and mild headaches. He had finished two tours in Vietnam several years previously and had had no previous medical illnesses.

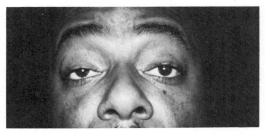

Upgaze

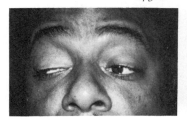 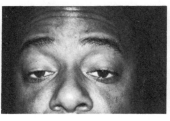

Right gaze   *Primary position*   *Left gaze*

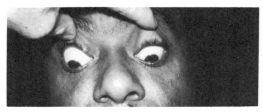

Downgaze

From R. W. Beck, et al. Melioidosis and bilateral third nerve palsy. Neurology *34:105, 1984. With permission.*

He had mild bilateral ptosis with limitation of elevation, depression, and adduction of each eye. A Tensilon test produced minimal improvement in motility. CT scan demonstrated enhancement in the interpeduncular fossa.

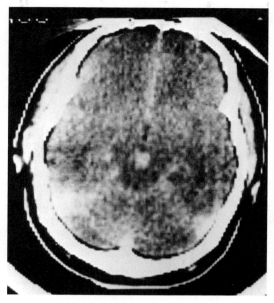

From R. W. Beck, et al. Melioidosis and bilateral third nerve palsy. Neurology *34:105, 1984. With permission.*

Because he was noted to have a temperature elevation to 103°F a lumbar puncture was performed. It demonstrated an elevated cell count and protein. He was ultimately found to have a central nervous system infection with *Pseudomonas pseudomallei,* which cleared completely with antibiotic therapy.

Central nervous system infections with a predilection for basal cistern pooling of inflammatory reaction may present with ophthalmoparesis, as in this case. Tuberculosis and meningococcal meningitis are the meningitides most likely to present with oculomotor disorders. The differential also includes sarcoidosis, carcinomatous meningitis, and fungal meningitides. When the underlying cause of an ophthalmoparesis is in doubt, CSF should be obtained to rule out a treatable disorder.

Möbius' Syndrome

A 23-year-old woman presented with symptoms of tunnel vision and headaches when her supervisor at work began to complain about her job performance. Her medical history was unknown with the exception of "a very traumatic birth."

On examination she had a complete horizontal ophthalmoplegia with full forced ductions. There was left facial weakness and deviation of the tongue (see below). A Tensilon test had negative results.

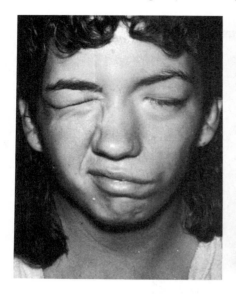 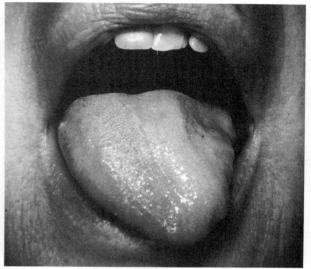

Visual field testing suggested functional constriction of the peripheral fields. Her neurologic examination disclosed mild retardation, unilateral tongue atrophy, and hyperactive deep tendon reflexes. CT scan of the posterior fossa demonstrated a small cystic structure in the interpeduncular fossa.

This patient has Möbius' syndrome, a congenital ophthalmoplegia associated with horizontal ophthalmoplegia, facial diplegia, tongue atrophy, and mild to moderate mental retardation. The absence of complaints referable to the ophthalmoparesis, coupled with the functional visual field deficit, were the tip-off that she had a long-standing (and benign) disorder.

Bibliography

Aarli, J. A. Oculopharyngeal muscular dystrophy. *Acta Neurol. Scand.* 45: 484, 1969.

Bastiaensen, L. A. K., et al. Ophthalmoplegia-plus, a real nosological entity. *Acta Neurol. Scand.* 58:9, 1978.

Bastiaensen, L. A. K., et al. Kearns syndrome or Kearns disease: Further evidence of a genuine entity in a case with uncommon features. *Ophthalmologica* 184:40, 1982.

Becker, W. J., Watters, G. V., and Humphreys, P. Fisher syndrome in childhood. *Neurology* 31:555, 1981.

Berenberg, R. A., et al. Lumping or splitting? "Ophthalmoplegia-plus" or Kearns-Sayre syndrome? *Ann. Neurol.* 1:37, 1977.

Fisher, C. M., and Adams, R. D. Diphtheritic polyneuritis: A pathological study. *J. Neuropathol. Exp. Neurol.* 15:243, 1956.

Fisher, M. An unusual variant of acute idiopathic polyneuritis (syndrome of ophthalmoplegia, ataxia and areflexia). *N. Engl. J. Med.* 255:57, 1956.

Kearns, T. P., and Sayre, G. P. Retinitis pigmentosa, external ophthalmoplegia, and complete heart block. *Arch. Ophthalmol.* 60:280, 1958.

Meienberg, O., and Ryffel, E. Supranuclear eye movement disorders in Fisher's syndrome of ophthalmoplegia, ataxia, and areflexia. *Arch. Neurol.* 40:402, 1983.

Mitsumoto, H., et al. Chronic progressive external ophthalmoplegia (CPEO): Clinical, morphologic, and biochemical studies. *Neurology* 33:452, 1983.

Murphy, S. F., and Drachman, D. B. The oculopharyngeal syndrome. *J.A.M.A.* 203:1003, 1968.

Sauron, B., et al. Miller Fisher syndrome: Clinical and electrophysiologic evidence of peripheral origin in 10 cases. *Neurology* 34:953, 1984.

Terranova, W., Palumbo, J. N., and Breman, J. G. Ocular findings in botulism type B. *J.A.M.A.* 241:475, 1979.

Van Allen, M. W., and Blodi, F. C. Neurologic aspects of the Möbius syndrome. *Neurology* 10:249, 1960.

Zasorin, N. L., Yee, R. D., and Baloh, R. W. Eye-movement abnormalities in ophthalmoplegia, ataxia, and areflexia: Fisher's syndrome. *Arch. Ophthalmol.* 103:55, 1985.

30

Orbital Apex Syndrome

A 48-year-old woman noted the abrupt onset of diplopia while driving. She had been seen by an acupuncturist 3 months earlier for left facial numbness. Two weeks previously she had noticed that the vision in her left eye appeared blurry.

Neuro-Ophthalmic Examination

	OD	OS
Visual acuity	20/20	20/100
Color plates correct	12 of 12	1 of 12
Pupils	Reverse relative afferent pupillary defect	6 mm (fixed)
Visual field	Normal	Central scotoma
Motility	Normal	Complete ophthalmoplegia
Orbits	Normal	Mild proptosis
Fundi	Normal	Normal

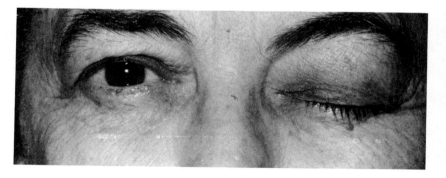

Results of a general neurologic examination were normal except for decreased sensation over the first trigeminal division on the left.

Summary

A middle-aged woman was found to have an internal and external ophthalmoplegia, visual field loss, impairment of first trigeminal division function, ptosis, and mild proptosis of the left eye.

Differential Diagnosis

The presence of unilateral involvement of the second, third, fourth, and fifth (first division) cranial nerves indicates a lesion in the region of the orbital apex. Further evidence of orbital apex involvement is the mild proptosis, which suggests either a mass behind the globe or blockage of the venous drainage system from the orbit.

Lesions anterior to the orbital apex would need to be massive to involve all of these structures, a feature not suggested by the mild proptosis. Lesions involving the anterior cavernous sinus might lead to a similar picture only without optic neuropathy.

Clinical Diagnosis: Orbital Apex Syndrome

The orbital apex contains the second, third, fourth, and fifth (first division) cranial nerves, as well as the sympathetic and parasympathetic innervation to the eye. The ophthalmic artery also traverses this region, as does a rich plexus of venous draining channels flowing from the orbit into the cavernous sinus.

The clinical distinction between the orbital apex and superior orbital fissure is more academic than pragmatic. Lesions involving this area may affect one or both structures with no clear demarcation between them and the anterior extension of the cavernous sinus. Because of the richness of the vascular supply, systemic diseases, metastatic lesions, and vascular anomalies may lead to orbital apex syndromes.

The gradual onset of orbital apex signs with or without associated pain in an adult suggests the presence of a metastatic lesion. In a middle-aged woman breast carcinoma has a predilection for this area. Scirrhous carcinoma of the breast leads to a characteristic retraction of the globe, while the other types of breast carcinoma present with mass effect, pain, and impaired cranial nerve function, as in the present patient. Other possibilities include meningioma, Graves' ophthalmopathy, orbital pseudotumor, and other types of metastatic disease.

Additional Testing

Neuroimaging of the orbital apex region should be performed. The radiologist should be directed to obtain coronal and axial views of this region with either computed tomography (CT) or magnetic resonance imaging (MRI). We have found CT scanning to be superior to MRI in this region for evaluation of bony involvement. If there is a suggestion of aneurysm on neuroimaging studies, arteriography should be carried out.

Whether or not a mass is visualized in an orbital apex or superior orbital fissure syndrome, a general medical evaluation, including chest x-ray, mammography (in the female patient), and serologic studies, should be done.

Management

With CT or MRI evidence of a mass in the orbital apex region, it is essential to look for other evidence of metastatic disease. If none is found and arteriography does not show an aneurysm then a biopsy for tissue diagnosis should be strongly considered.

Management and Course of the Case

CT scan demonstrated a mass in the region of the left orbital apex with contiguous bony changes.

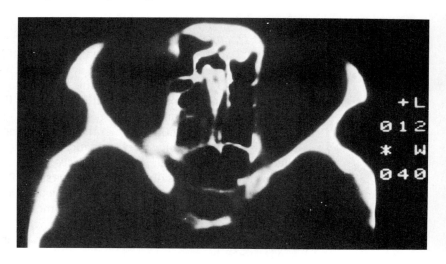

The patient was noted to have a mass on breast examination. Biopsy and modified radical mastectomy were carried out; the tumor was found histologically to be a mucinous carcinoma. Her left orbital apex region was radiated, with complete clearing of her findings over a 4-week period.

Tolosa-Hunt Syndrome

A 32-year-old flight attendant noted diplopia and a painful left eye on a trans-Pacific flight. The pain was described as "excruciating," having come on over a 5-hour period. His medical history was otherwise unremarkable. On examination he had left ptosis with limitation of the left eye on upgaze, adduction, and abduction. Downgaze was normal (see below). Funduscopic findings were unremarkable, and his visual acuity and pupillary function were normal. CT scan and results of cerebrospinal fluid studies were normal. Within hours of the oral administration of prednisone 60 mg, his pain abated, with clearing of the motility deficits and ptosis over a 5-day period. At 1 year after cessation of therapy he remains asymptomatic.

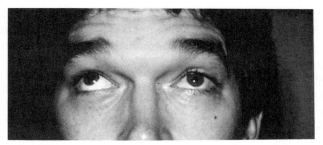

Upgaze

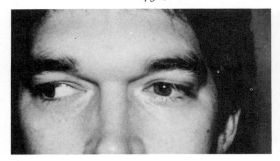

Right gaze

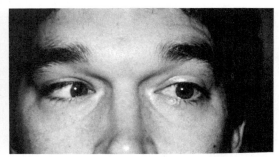

Left gaze

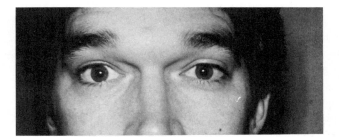

Primary position

This patient's painful ophthalmoplegia exemplifies the superior orbital fissure syndrome, a posterior orbit, anterior cavernous sinus idiopathic inflammatory process (Tolosa-Hunt syndrome, orbital pseudotumor). This is usually a benign, self-limiting disease without known cause. Women are affected more commonly than men, and it is more prevalent in blacks than whites. The Tolosa-Hunt syndrome can affect any aspect of the cavernous sinus or orbital region; its diagnosis is based on the exclusion of other diseases and the clinical response to corticosteroids. This diagnosis always should make the clinician uncomfortable as underlying diseases not infrequently surface later.

The evaluation of a painful ophthalmoplegia includes directed neuroimaging of the orbit and cavernous sinus regions. If neuroimaging results are normal, a course of corticosteroids should be carefully begun, with follow-up neuroimaging if the pain or ophthalmoplegia is refractory to the treatment. In the patient over 60 years of age, an erythrocyte sedimentation rate should be obtained to rule out the possibility of giant cell arteritis.

Bibliography

Holt, H., and de Rotth, A. Orbital apex and sphenoid fissure syndrome. *Arch. Ophthalmol.* 24:731, 1940.

Kline, L. B. The Tolosa-Hunt syndrome. *Surv. Ophthalmol.* 27:79, 1982.

Schatz, N. J. Pain Associated with Ophthalmoplegia. *N.O.A.O. Symposium on Neuro-ophthalmology.* St. Louis: Mosby, 1976. Pp. 73–79.

31

Myasthenia Gravis

A 74-year-old man noted difficulty reading his evening newspaper, complaining, "My eyelid gets in the way." He also reported horizontal diplopia with extended reading. He had no other symptoms and was not taking medication.

Neuro-Ophthalmic Examination

	OD	OS
Visual acuity	20/20	20/20
Color plates correct	10 of 10	10 of 10
Pupils	Normal	Normal
Motility	Normal	Normal
Fundi	Normal	Normal
Visual field	Normal	Normal

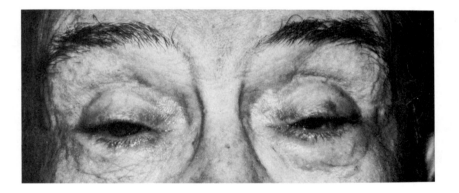

Results of a neurologic examination were normal.

Summary
An elderly man was found to have bilateral ptosis.

Differential Diagnosis
Lesions causing bilateral ptosis may involve the levator muscles, neuro-muscular junctions, third cranial nerves, or midbrain region. The absence of other brainstem findings on examination, coupled with a lack of

sensory findings or pupillary involvement, mitigates against involvement of brainstem or third nerve. The history is not suggestive of a primary myopathy (see Chapter 29). Fatigable ptosis that is bilateral and associated with other evidence of ophthalmoparesis should always bring to mind the diagnosis of myasthenia gravis.

Clinical Diagnosis: Myasthenia Gravis

Myasthenia gravis is an immunologically mediated disorder that involves the binding of antibodies to striate muscle acetylcholine receptor protein in such a way as to block the normal synaptic transmission of a neurochemical agent (acetylcholine) to the muscle membrane. This disease commonly affects the extraocular muscles: Fifty percent of patients present with ocular symptoms, and over 90 percent eventually develop eye movement abnormalities.

Ocular myasthenia refers to myasthenia limited to the eyes on clinical examination. This involvement may often be asymmetric or localized and mimic third (clinically, pupil-spared), fourth, or sixth cranial nerve palsy; gaze paresis; internuclear ophthalmoplegia (INO); or other strabismus. The hallmark of ocular myasthenia is the fatigability of lid function on sustained upward or lateral gaze positions.

Pure ocular myasthenia gravis presents no risk to life and only moderate disability. However, as noted below, the ocular symptoms may be quite resistant to treatment despite dramatic short-lived responses to parenteral Tensilon employed for diagnosis. The natural history of ocular myasthenia is not fully known. When systemic involvement occurs, it generally becomes symptomatic within 2 years of the onset of the ocular involvement. In approximately 40 percent of patients presenting with eye signs alone, systemic disease is never manifested. The identification of patients at risk of proceeding to generalized disease from the ocular form is, at best, speculative.

Careful analysis of saccadic movements and fixation in patients with ocular myasthenia has identified specific findings that can assist clinicians in earlier recognition of the neuromuscular nature of the disease process. Saccades of normal velocity, despite limited range of movement, are characteristic of myasthenia. This contrasts with a paretic process such as a nerve palsy, in which saccades in the direction of the limited duction are slowed.

The quick phases of optokinetic nystagmus (OKN) may be slowed with repeated passes of the OKN tape or drum, and sustained extremes of gaze may lead to increasing nystagmus; these latter two findings may lead to the appearance of a pseudo-INO in ocular myasthenia, with slowness of the adducting saccade and nystagmus of the abducting eye. Other findings include rapid small saccades with a "quiver" at the end of the movement leading to what have been called lighteninglike saccades and saccadic dysmetria. Many of these findings will clear with the administration of Tensilon, as outlined below.

Other findings helpful in the clinical diagnosis of ocular myasthenia include the presence of "lid twitch," a transient eyelid retraction during refixations from down to straight ahead, and a "curtain sign" (when the ptotic eyelid is elevated manually, the normal-appearing eyelid settles into more of a ptotic position).

Additional Testing

Any ptosis, oculomotor disturbance, or gaze paresis without obvious explanation should be investigated for the possibility of myasthenia. The intravenous administration of Tensilon is the diagnostic procedure of choice in establishing this diagnosis. Tensilon, a short-acting inhibitor of acetylcholinesterase, effectively increases the amount of acetylcholine at the postsynaptic receptor site where more of this neurotransmitter is required to create muscle contraction in myasthenia. Longer-acting anticholinesterase agents can also be used for diagnostic testing. The various types of tests are described below.

TENSILON TEST

Tensilon is supplied in single-dose, 10-mg/ml, break-neck vials. A 1-ml tuberculin syringe works well for determining the exact amount injected.

The following materials are needed for a Tensilon test:

1. Tensilon 10 mg (before expiration date)
2. Atropine 0.4 mg
3. Injectable saline
4. Tuberculin syringe
5. 10-ml syringe (for saline injection)
6. 21-gauge needle
7. Camera (optional)

A specific end point—a specific amount of ptosis or degree of oculomotor or gaze paresis—should be determined before administering Tensilon. The end point should not consist of the subjective response of the patient. If possible, photographs of the patient should be taken before and after the administration of Tensilon to document the degree of response and to prevent multiple tests to satisfy the observer of the diagnosis.

The side effects of Tensilon include an increase in bronchial secretion, bradycardia, bronchospasm, nausea, and weakness; any of these may be severe if the patient is hypersensitive to acetylcholinesterase. For this reason, many clinicians prefer to give atropine 0.4 mg either intramuscularly 15 minutes before, or intravenously immediately before Tensilon testing. We generally pretreat with 0.3 to 0.4 mg of atropine intravenously immediately before the test, keeping an additional 0.6 mg of this preparation on hand for any untoward side effects.

A small-bore (21-gauge or less) needle is inserted into either a dorsal hand or antecubital vein, ensuring that venous blood can be withdrawn to establish that it is within the vein.

Tensilon 2 mg (0.2 ml in the 1-ml tuberculin syringe) is then injected as a test dose, using a small amount of injectable saline to flush the Tensilon into the vein. (Frequently this amount of Tensilon gives the desired result of increased movement or lessened ptosis, and the diagnosis is made.) If no response occurs in 1 to 2 minutes of observation, then an additional 8 mg (0.8 ml) is slowly injected, followed by another saline flush. The response, if any, should be recorded photographically and the patient put in the supine position if any bradycardia is present.

NEOSTIGMINE BROMIDE (PROSTIGMIN) TEST

Neostigmine bromide (Prostigmin), a longer-acting anticholinesterase agent, can be given as an intramuscular injection (0.5–1.0 mg). The onset of action of Prostigmin may be 15 to 30 minutes from the time of injection, and the action may last several hours. Intramuscular atropine, 0.4 mg, is given 15 to 20 minutes before the test injection. The patient should be observed closely for a response (or side effects) during the onset of peak action of this medication. This test is particularly useful in children or uncooperative adults.

ACETYLCHOLINE RECEPTOR ANTIBODY TITER

The serum of 70 to 90 percent of patients with myasthenia gravis will have antibodies to acetylcholine receptor. In purely ocular myasthenia, the presence of an elevated titer drops to less than 10 percent. Although this test may be helpful when a high titer is present, absence of these antibodies doe not rule out ocular myasthenia.

ELECTRODIAGNOSTIC STUDIES

Repetitive Nerve Stimulation. The repetitive electrical stimulation of muscle in a myasthenic patient will produce a characteristic decrement in the amplitude of the muscle electrical response, compared with a normal control. This finding is helpful in the diagnosis of the patient with suspected generalized myasthenia, and it may or may not be present in the ocular myasthenic.

Single-Fiber Electromyogram. Single-fiber electromyogram (SFEMG) allows the recording of extracellular action potentials from single muscle fibers within a given motor unit. The presence of variability between individual muscle fibers suggests a difference in rapidity of neuromuscular transmission between fibers, a finding seen in myasthenics. Abnormal SFEMG, however, is seen in other neurogenic diseases and is not specific for myasthenia.

Curariform Drug Tests. The application of curarelike agents to the postsynaptic membrane of a normal muscle will lead to a blockade of acetylcholine receptors. In myasthenics, in whom there is already a partial blockade of the acetylcholine receptor sites, an increased sensitivity to curariform drugs is seen. This response can be quantified by either systemic or regional curarization. An increased sensitivity further confirms the diagnosis of myasthenia gravis.

RADIOLOGIC TESTING
In the patient with suspected or confirmed myasthenia gravis, computed tomography (CT) or magnetic resonance imaging (MRI) of the chest will best assess the possibility of thymoma. Lymphoepithelial thymoma is present in 10 to 15 percent of patients with myasthenia gravis.

Treatment

The treatment of myasthenia gravis involves either replenishing acetylcholine at the motor end-plate or decreasing the blockade induced by the receptor-antibody binding. The neuromuscular blockade can be overcome by the administration of acetylcholinesterase-inhibiting agents that increase the supply of acetylcholine at the receptor site. The immunologic response can be blocked with corticosteroids or chemotherapy, or by removing the immunologic factors by thymectomy or plasmapheresis.

The treatment of ocular myasthenia depends on the severity of the disease. Mild bilateral or unilateral ptosis may not require treatment if there is no inconvenience to the patient. In cases in which the ptosis is an inconvenience or there is accompanying ophthalmoplegia or generalized myasthenia, we initiate treatment with oral pyridostigmine bromide (Mestinon) 30 mg twice daily, gradually increasing the dosage to tolerance or clinical response. Not infrequently, however, the acetylcholinesterase inhibitors are ineffective in treating ocular myasthenia.

In symptomatic ocular myasthenia unresponsive to Mestinon, we have often seen dramatic responses to the oral administration of corticosteroids. When corticosteroids are indicated, we initiate treatment with prednisone in a daily dose of 80 to 100 mg, tapering to an alternate-day dosage after 1 to 2 weeks. Although high-dose corticosteroids have been found to exacerbate generalized myasthenia initially, leading to generalized weakness and in some cases respiratory compromise, this is an infrequent occurrence (never in our experience) in ocular myasthenia. Whether or not hospitalization is required during the initiation of corticosteroid therapy is controversial.

In the otherwise healthy patient (and certainly in the patient with a thymoma) with symptomatic generalized myasthenia gravis unresponsive to Mestinon or corticosteroids, thymectomy should be considered. Other treatments to remove the circulating antibodies to receptor protein are well reviewed elsewhere and beyond the scope of this book.

Often, purely ocular myasthenia will not respond to the conventional treatments, and the patient is left with diplopia or ptosis. If the patient has no generalized signs or symptoms it is best not to push potentially harmful treatments to attempt control of the ocular involvement. In these individuals, lid crutches or taping may be of benefit.

Management and Course of the Case

A Tensilon test was carried out, confirming the diagnosis of myasthenia.

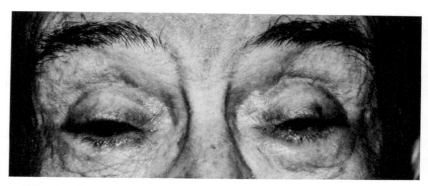

Eyelid position before administration of Tensilon.

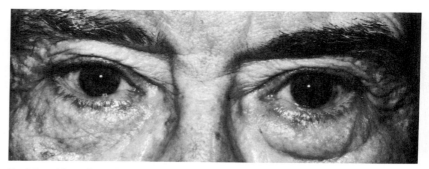

Eyelid position after administration of Tensilon.

Chest CT scan demonstrated an invasive thymoma, which was removed surgically, and postoperative irradiation was performed. Subsequently, the patient did well on a regimen of Mestinon and corticosteroids with complete clearing of his ptosis and symptoms of diplopia. He died of pulmonary extension of the thymoma, an unusual occurrence.

Ptosis—Myasthenia Gravis

A 28-year-old man complained of intermittent diplopia and eyelid "drooping" while playing squash. He had no other relevant medical history. Examination showed left-sided ptosis with full motility. Tensilon testing was carried out after the intravenous administration of 0.3 mg of atropine. This produced prompt resolution of the ptosis. The patient remains asymptomatic on a regimen of Mestinon 60 mg four times daily.

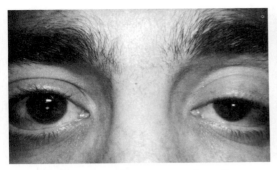

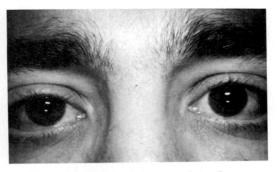

Eyelid position before administration of Tensilon.   *Eyelid position after administration of Tensilon.*

This case represents a relatively straightforward case of ocular myasthenia. The fatigable nature of the ptosis and concurrence of ocular motility symptoms suggested involvement of the neuromuscular junction. In our experience, roughly one-half of patients with ocular myasthenia have a good initial response to Mestinon.

Senile Ptosis

A 68-year-old woman was referred for evaluation of ptosis, which she had noted over the preceding 2-year period.

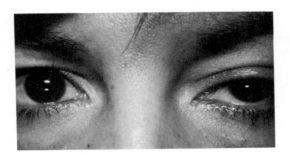

Results of her examination were normal except for the ptosis. She had full extraocular motility and normal pupillary responses. A Tensilon test had negative results. Old photographs showed that she had had the ptosis for at least 20 years. Because the lid droop was cosmetically bothersome, she was referred to an oculoplastics specialist for surgical correction.

"Senile" ptosis is an isolated ptosis in the elderly that is not congenital and represents a disinsertion or dehiscence of the levator aponeurosis. Generally, no treatment is necessary, although if obstructing vision or cosmetically unacceptable, the lids can be raised surgically.

Congenital Ptosis

A 7-year-old boy was referred for evaluation of right-sided ptosis. His mother had noted an asymmetry of the eyelids since birth. On examination 4 to 5 mm of ptosis was noted on the right. Minimal limitation of elevation was also noted on the same side. Visual acuity, pupils, fundi, and orbicularis oculi function were normal.

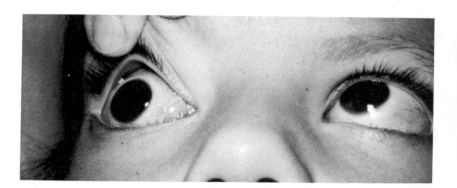

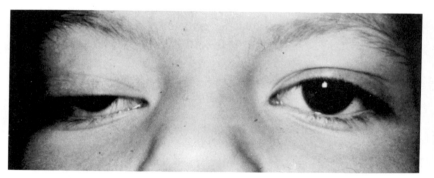

Primary position

Photographs taken at the time of birth showed a ptosis. This child has a congenital ptosis, which may be isolated or associated with limitation in elevation of the ipsilateral eye (as in this case). Any ptosis of unexplained causation mandates obtaining old photographs for review. Often the basis of the ptosis is uncovered by looking at these photos with magnification, thereby obviating further potentially dangerous and costly testing.

Bilateral Ptosis from Brainstem Lesion

A 24-year-old man noted droopy eyelids and vertical diplopia, which became worse over a 1-month period. Results of a neuro-ophthalmic examination were normal except for bilateral ptosis and 4 diopters of left hypertropia on right gaze. Motility and pupillary responses were otherwise normal, as were results of a general neurologic exam.

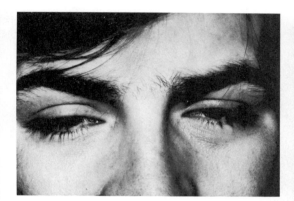
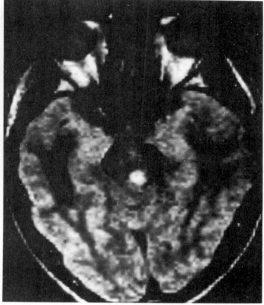

MRI showed a mass in the region of the third nerve nucleus. Although a histologic diagnosis was not obtained, the mass was presumed to be a brainstem glioma.

Although extremely rare, selective lesions of the brainstem oculomotor nuclei and supranuclear pathways mediating lid function may lead to bilateral or, very rarely, unilateral ptosis. Other evidence of contiguous central nervous system involvement should, however, be present. We routinely obtain MRI studies of all patients with nonneuromuscular bilateral ptosis of progressive onset. This noninvasive tool has the best yield for defining brainstem pathology.

A local television anchorman received several phone calls about a droop of his left eyelid. He had had a recent severe migraine headache requiring intramuscular narcotic analgesics. There was no history of neck trauma or other systemic medical symptoms.

Old photographs were obtained, showing that the ptosis and anisocoria had not been present 1 year previously.

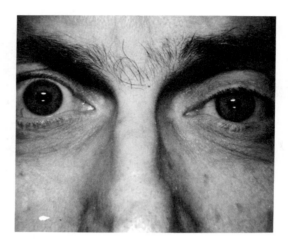

Instillation of hydroxyamphetamine hydrobromide (Paredrine) resulted in no perceptible dilation, which suggested a postganglionic basis for the oculosympathetic paresis.

This man has an oculosympathetic paresis, or Horner's syndrome. The sympathetic pathway to the dilator muscle of the iris is composed of three neurons: The first two neurons extend from the cervical cord out along the apex of the lung to synapse at the bifurcation of the carotid artery. The last neuron travels up the internal carotid to enter the orbit with the ophthalmic artery (see Fig. 1-19).

The diagnostic evaluation of Horner's syndrome is discussed in Chapters 1 and 33. Results of the Paredrine test in this case are consistent with an oculosympathetic paresis resulting from injury to the carotid sheath during the migraine attack. Evaluation of an oculosympathetic paresis in patients over the age of 50 years should carefully exclude second-order neuron involvement from lung and spinal cord lesions.

Bibliography

Bever, C. T., et al. Prognosis of ocular myasthenia. *Neurology* 30:387, 1980.

Cogan, D. G. Myasthenia gravis: A review of the disease and a description of lid twitch as a characteristic sign. *Arch. Ophthalmol.* 74:217, 1965.

Conway, V. H., et al. Isolated bilateral complete ptosis. *Can. J. Ophthalmol.* 18 : 37, 1983.

Daroff, R. B. Ocular Myasthenia: Diagnosis and Therapy. In J. S. Glaser (ed.), *Neuro-ophthalmology Symposium of the University of Miami and the Bascom Palmer Eye Institute.* St. Louis: Mosby, 1980. Vol. 10, p. 62.

Dortzbach, R. K., and Sutula, F. C. Involutional blepharoptosis: A histopathological study. *Arch. Ophthalmol.* 98 : 2045, 1980.

Lisak, R. P., and Barchi, R. L. *Myasthenia Gravis (Major Problems in Neurology,* Vol. 11). Philadelphia: Saunders, 1982.

Miller, N. R., Morris, J. E., and Maguire, M. Combined use of neostigmine and ocular motility measurements in the diagnosis of myasthenia gravis. *Arch. Ophthalmol.* 100 : 761, 1982.

Spooner, J. W., and Baloh, R. W. Eye movement fatigue in myasthenia gravis. *Neurology* 29 : 29, 1979.

32

Lid Retraction

A 23-year-old woman was noted by her husband to have "widened eyes." She had noted increasing fatigue over the previous 6 months but had no focal symptoms.

Neuro-Ophthalmic Examination

	OD	OS
Visual acuity	20/20	20/20
Color plates correct	10 of 10	10 of 10
Visual field	Normal	Normal
Fundi	Normal	Normal
Motility	Normal	Normal
Pupils	Normal	Normal

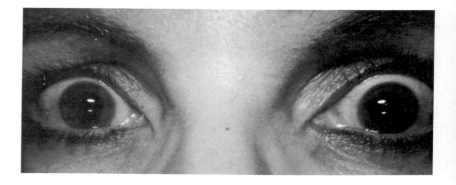

Summary

A young adult was noted to have asymptomatic lid retraction.

Differential Diagnosis

The upper lid normally covers the superior limbus by 1 to 2 mm. When sclera is seen between the superior limbus and the upper lid, lid retraction is present. The causes of lid retraction are:

1. Dysthyroid orbitopathy
2 Midbrain lid retraction (Collier's sign)
3. Volitional lid retraction
4. Nondysthyroid cicatricial retraction
5. Pseudo—lid retraction with contralateral ptosis in myasthenia gravis

When the lid retraction is present in primary position and downgaze, it is usually due to cicatricial retraction (alteration of the lid tissues themselves) related to the dysthyroid state. The retraction seen with Collier's sign does not persist in downgaze. Volitional retraction is characterized by the presence of a furrowed brow from the patient's attempts to keep the eyelids open further than normal.

Clinical Diagnosis: Dysthyroid Lid Retraction
The occurrence of lid retraction in dysthyroid orbitopathy has no relationship to the state of the thyroid function. It may be seen in the hyperthyroid, euthyroid, or hypothyroid states. Its presence may improve or persist after the hyperthyroid state is successfully treated.

Treatment
The indications for treatment of dysthyroid lid retraction are either corneal exposure or cosmetic. Surgical treatment should not be performed until the underlying orbitopathy or endocrine imbalance has been quiescent for a considerable period (at least 6 months).

Management and Course of the Case
The patient was found to be hyperthyroid and was treated medically. The lid retraction gradually improved over a 1-month period.

Pseudo—Lid Retraction in Myasthenia

A 60-year-old man noted intermittent diplopia and was referred for further evaluation because of lid retraction. His history was otherwise relevant only for difficulty chewing solid foods. Ocular motility testing showed abduction deficits in both eyes, with retraction of the left lid present only in primary position and accompanied by furrowing of the brows. When the left eye was covered, the right upper lid assumed a ptotic position.

This finding indicates that the patient has pseudo—lid retraction from volitional attempts to keep his right eyelid open. When he was given Tensilon, his eye findings resolved, which confirmed the diagnosis of myasthenia (see Chapter 31).

33

Horner's Syndrome

When a 55-year-old man had one of his usually severe left-sided migraines, he noted a drooping of his left eyelid and a large right pupil. There was no history of neck manipulation, and he was in otherwise excellent health.

Neuro-Ophthalmic Examination

	OD	OS
Visual acuity	20/20	20/20
Color plates correct	10 of 10	10 of 10
Motility	Normal	Normal
Fundi	Normal	Normal
Pupils (in light)	4 mm	3 mm
(in dark)	7 mm	4 mm

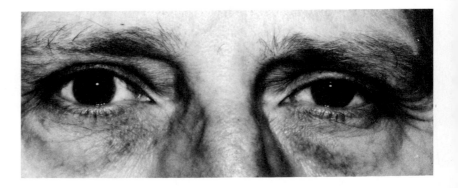

Results of neurologic and medical examinations were normal.

Summary
A 55-year-old man was noted to have ptosis and anisocoria (greater in darkness) after a migraine attack.

Differential Diagnosis

Since the anisocoria was greater in dim than bright illumination, the abnormality was in the left pupil. Miosis associated with ipsilateral ptosis indicates damage to the sympathetic innervation to the eye and defines the entity Horner's syndrome (oculosympathetic paresis).

The ptosis of Horner's syndrome is best evaluated with the patient upright with the gravitational effect on the lid; a patient lying in bed may not exhibit a clinically noticeable ptosis. The miosis is best evaluated in both dim and bright lighting to determine if there is a dilation lag in darkness characteristic of an oculosympathetic paresis. These patients are best examined when not emotionally distraught; an anxious patient may paradoxically dilate the miotic pupil of a Horner's syndrome greater than its fellow eye because of postdenervation hypersensitivity and an increase in circulating epinephrine.

Clinical Diagnosis: Oculosympathetic Paresis (Horner's Syndrome)

The sympathetic innervation of the iris sphincter derives from a chain of three neurons. A rudimentary knowledge of the course of these neurons is useful in determining the clinical importance of an oculosympathetic paresis (see Fig. 1-19).

The first-order neuron originates in the hypothalamic region, traveling through the brainstem in the reticular system and the intermediolateral cell column of the cervical spinal cord. The second-order neuron originates between the spinal levels of C8 and T1, exiting the spinal cord here to travel cephalad along the vertebral column adjacent to the apex of the lung and joining the common carotid artery in the neck. The final neuron in the chain originates near the carotid bifurcation after giving off sympathetic fibers to the face that travel along the external carotid artery. The oculosympathetic fibers then travel with the internal carotid through the cavernous sinus and enter the orbit through the superior orbital fissure.

The oculosympathetic input to the eye stimulates iris pigmentation, with the coloration of the iris fixed after age 2 to 3 years. Lesions involving this system before this age may lead to heterochromia iridis, a clinical finding important in the determination of causation.

Damage to any of the three neurons in the oculosympathetic pathway lead to the following findings:

1. Miosis
2. Ptosis (both upper and lower lid)
3. Apparent enophthalmos
4. Increase in accommodative amplitude
5. Heterochromia iridis (congenital Horner's syndrome)
6. Decreased tear production
7. Facial anhidrosis (when first- or second-order neuron is affected)

The evaluation of an oculosympathetic paresis should be aimed at determining the site of involvement along the three-order neuronal arc. Lesions affecting the first-order neuron typically have accompanying signatures of neurologic compromise, and these are usually obvious on even a cursory neurologic examination. The important distinction, therefore, is between lesions of the second-order and third-order neurons. Lesions affecting the second neuron in the chain are found along the vertebral bodies or within the apex of the lung. These tend to be either tumor or trauma affecting the cervical spine. Lesions affecting the last neuron in the chain are usually vascular, affecting the carotid artery or the vascular plexus within the cavernous sinus. Common causes of Horner's syndrome are:

I. First-order neuron
   A. Stroke (brainstem)
   B. Trauma
   C. Spinal cord tumors
II. Second-order neuron
   A. Trauma (neck)
   B. Vertebral metastases
   C. Apical lung lesions
III. Third-order neuron
   A. Migraine
   B. Carotid trauma
      1. Iatrogenic (from old method of angiography)
      2. Neck manipulation
   C. Dissecting carotid aneurysm
   D. Cavernous sinus lesion

Additional Testing

We recommend the use of cocaine eyedrops if the diagnosis of a Horner's syndrome cannot be made clinically. Cocaine (4–10%) should be instilled in both eyes, and the pupillary diameters measured under similar lighting conditions at 30 minutes. Cocaine blocks the reuptake of norepinephrine by the postganglionic nerve fibers; its instillation in an eye with any of the three-neuron chain dysfunctional will lead to either reduced or no pupillary dilation in the affected eye since there is impairment of the stimulation to release this chemical. The patient's other eye acts as a control, testing the efficacy of the cocaine preparation. This test merely confirms the existence of oculosympathetic paresis but does not provide information about the site of the lesion.

The distinction between second- and third-order neuron Horner's syndrome is best determined by the use of the hydroxyamphetamine hydrobromide (Paredrine) test. Paredrine 1% is instilled in both eyes, and the pupillary diameters are observed under similar lighting conditions 45 minutes later. Paredrine acts to release norepinephrine from the sympathetic granules at the presynaptic terminal and will dilate the pupil when the third-order neuron is intact. If the suspect pupil does not dilate, or does so only partially, then the sympathetic postganglionic (third-order) neuron is the culprit. Again, the normal pupil should act as the control, testing the efficacy of the Paredrine preparation. Involvement of the third-order (postganglionic) neuron is seen in neck trauma, iatrogenic causes (old method of arteriography via direct carotid puncture), migraine with ischemia of the carotid sympathetic chain, or disease in the cavernous sinus or orbit. Cases of postganglionic oculosympathetic paresis should be evaluated with a careful history and by observing old photographs. If the finding has occurred within the past 3 years and there is no history of neck trauma or migraine, then the patient should be closely followed. Neuroimaging of the orbits and cavernous sinus should be obtained if other symptoms or neurologic findings develop. If the postganglionic oculosympathetic paresis is of abrupt onset in an individual over the age of 50 with ipsilateral unrelenting neck or head pain, a cerebral arteriogram should be obtained to rule out a dissecting carotid aneurysm.

The absence of accompanying neurologic findings in a patient with Horner's syndrome, coupled with dilation of the involved pupil with Paredrine, suggests second-order oculosympathetic involvement. It is in the pathway of the second-order neuron that primary or secondary lung tumors or vertebral metastases can lead to oculosympathetic paresis. In these patients, evaluation should include a chest x-ray with apical lordotic views and cervical spine films. If these are normal, then the patient should be followed closely for the development of an underlying malignancy.

The importance of obtaining a patient's old photographs cannot be overemphasized; the presence of a Horner's syndrome for more than 2 years is convincing evidence that the process is a benign one, even without extensive testing.

Treatment

The treatment of this affliction should be aimed at the underlying disease, of which the Horner's syndrome is but a manifestation. Once the presence of Horner's syndrome has been established, the involved order in the neuronal chain determined, and the duration of its presence documented by old photographs, then one is armed with the information necessary to follow the patient. The ptosis of oculosympathetic paresis is usually asymptomatic, although ptosis surgery provides a good cosmetic effect in the patient bothered by the appearance of the lid droop.

Management and Course of the Case

Paredrine testing demonstrated no dilation of the involved pupil, suggesting third-order (postganglionic) oculosympathetic nerve involvement. This is consistent with damage to the sympathetic chain along the carotid sheath from the vasospasm of migraine. The patient was treated with a beta blocker and has remained headache free for 1 year. The ptosis and miosis have remained unchanged.

Horner's Syndrome in a Child

A 3-year-old boy was noted to have anisocoria after minor head trauma. At the age of 6 months he had had spinal surgery for a tumor that was removed from his neck region.

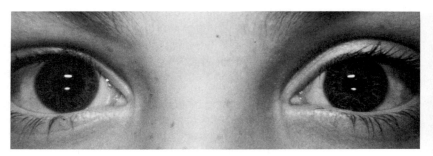

The presence of the heterochromia accompanying this oculosympathetic paresis underscores its early age of onset. Paredrine testing and general neurologic examination suggested the presence of second-order neuron involvement, consistent with trauma to the sympathetic chain in the cervical region where the tumor had been removed. No further evaluation was considered necessary.

As mentioned in the previous case, the presence of heterochromia iridis (or photographic evidence of duration of more than 2 to 3 years) in a patient with "newly discovered" Horner's syndrome is reassurance that no progressive disorder exists.

Bibliography
Giles, C. L., and Henderson, J. W. Horner's syndrome: An analysis of 216 cases. *Am. J. Ophthalmol.* 46:289, 1958.

Grimson, B. S., and Thompson, H. S. Raeder's syndrome: A clinical review. *Surv. Ophthalmol.* 24:199, 1980.

Maloney, W. F., Younge, B. R., and Moyer, N. J. Evaluation of the causes and accuracy of pharmacologic localization in Horner's syndrome. *Am. J. Ophthalmol.* 90:394, 1980.

Thompson, H. S., and Mensher, J. H. Adrenergic mydriasis in Horner's syndrome: Hydroxyamphetamine test for diagnosis of postganglionic defects. *Am. J. Ophthalmol.* 72:472, 1971.

Thompson, H. S., and Pilley, S. F. J. Unequal pupils: A flow chart for sorting out the anisocorias. *Surv. Ophthalmol.* 21:45, 1976.

Weinstein, J. M., Zweifel, T. J., and Thompson, H. S. Congenital Horner's syndrome. *Arch. Ophthalmol.* 98:1074, 1980.

34

Dilated Pupil—Adie's Syndrome

A 34-year-old woman noted blurred vision in the right eye, and when a computed tomography (CT) scan of her head was found to be normal she was referred for neuro-ophthalmic examination.

Neuro-Ophthalmic Examination

	OU
Visual acuity	20/20
Color plates correct	12 of 12
Visual field	Normal
Fundi	Normal
Motility	Normal

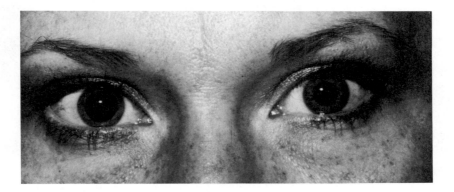

Results of a neurologic examination were normal.

Summary

A young woman was found to have a fixed, dilated pupil, with normal ocular motility and otherwise normal results on neurologic examination.

Differential Diagnosis

As with any anisocoria, it is first necessary to decide if the pathologic pupil is the larger or the smaller of the pair. A discussion of how to examine the pupil is included in Chapter 1. A fixed dilated pupil, in the absence of ocular motility disturbance, is usually from iris trauma, Adie's syndrome, or pharmacologic blockade. A third nerve palsy could theoretically present initially with just pupillary involvement and no ptosis or extraocular motility disturbance, but this is extremely rare. Unilateral pupillary dilation can occur during migraine, but this is transient and usually without residual deficit. There was no obvious evidence of old iris trauma on external examination of this patient's eyes. The major differential diagnosis for the otherwise asymptomatic unreactive pupil is between Adie's syndrome and pharmacologic blockade.

The pilocarpine test readily distinguishes parasympathetic denervation from pharmacologic blockade. In the latter, 1% pilocarpine cannot overcome the postsynaptic receptor blockade, and the pupil remains dilated. An unreactive pupil from third nerve paresis will constrict briskly to 1% pilocarpine, as will an Adie's pupil. A nonacute Adie's pupil will usually constrict to 0.1% pilocarpine, since denervation supersensitivity will be present. See Fig. 1-20 for a flowchart on the testing of the abnormal pupil.

In this patient, dilute pilocarpine promptly constricted the dilated pupil (see below), suggesting a lesion involving, or distal to, the ciliary ganglion and confirming the diagnosis of Adie's or tonic pupil.

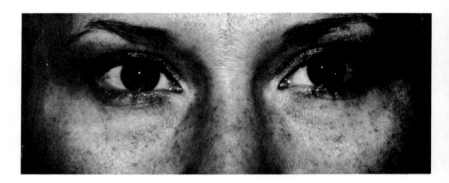

Clinical Diagnosis: Adie's Pupil (Tonic Pupil)

Adie's syndrome is seen most frequently in women between the ages of 20 and 40 years. These patients present either having just noticed that they have a dilated pupil or complaining of poor accommodation or light sensitivity. When first seen these patients have a dilated pupil that does not respond to direct light or exhibit the near response. Denervation supersensitivity to dilute pilocarpine may not be present acutely. Within days, the pupil will regain some of the near response and demonstrate the characteristic denervation supersensitivity to pilocarpine. On slit lamp examination at this time, sectors of the iris that have no contraction are seen, while other sectors respond sluggishly to light, giving the iris the appearance of *vermiform contractions*. These sectorial palsies are due to scattered involvement of the postganglionic fibers and are a hallmark of the entity. Over a period of years, the pupil will become smaller. The findings of tonic pupil constriction to near greater than the response to light—plus sectorial iris palsies—establish the clinical diagnosis of Adie's syndrome. The dilute pilocarpine test can then be used for confirmation.

When the patient with a tonic pupil is found to have diminished or absent deep tendon reflexes (which may be asymmetric in reactivity—like the iris involvement), the condition is referred to as the Holmes-Adie syndrome. On close questioning, a large number of these patients report that they also have symptoms of asymmetric sweating or constipation, which suggest more diffuse autonomic nervous system involvement.

Initially, both pupils may be involved in Adie's syndrome (10%). Unilateral cases become bilateral at a rate of 4 percent per year. When involvement of the other eye occurs several years later, there is a prominent anisocoria, with the older tonic pupil smaller than the new. Over many years, both pupils will become smaller and nonreactive to light, a finding that may make distinction from Argyll Robertson pupils difficult.

Treatment

There is no treatment for Adie's syndrome. The identification of the tonic pupil is crucial, however, in halting unnecessary (and potentially harmful) neurodiagnostic testing. Occasionally, for cosmetic purposes, dilute pilocarpine may be prescribed to even up the size of the pupils. However, the side effects of the pilocarpine, including blurred vision and pain, are usually greater than any benefit from this type of treatment. In those patients bothered by the accommodative difficulties, reading glasses are helpful.

Management and Course of the Case

The patient continued to have symptoms of glare when entering bright lighting, in addition to vague symptoms of leg dysesthesias and mild constipation. Two years after the diagnosis of her right tonic pupil, the left became involved, and her neurologic examination showed depressed reflexes in the legs.

Dilated Pupil—Pharmacologic

A 23-year-old nurse presented to an emergency room with a severe left-sided headache and dilated pupil. After CT scan, lumbar puncture results, and cerebral angiogram were found to be normal, she was referred for neuro-ophthalmic evaluation. Pilocarpine (1%) was placed in her eyes and failed to constrict the involved pupil. The patient's belongings were searched, and a bottle of atropine drops was found. She was referred for psychiatric evaluation.

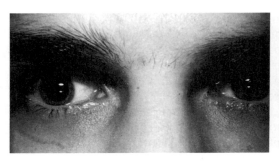

Before administration of 1% pilocarpine.

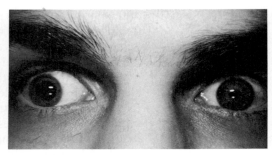

After administration of 1% pilocarpine.

The "toxic" pupil is a result of pharmacologic agents' altering pupillary size by action on the central or peripheral nervous system. When the action is systemic, the pupils are involved symmetrically. In this patient's case, the action was a direct paralysis of the parasympathetic fibers to the iris by atropine, which could not be overcome by the pilocarpine. Similarly, inadvertent dilation may occur when pharmacologic agents are unknowingly rubbed into the eye. This may be seen in individuals who have placed scopolamine patches behind one ear for prevention of motion sickness.

Dilated Pupils from Dopamine Hydrochloride

A 58-year-old patient in the coronary care unit was noted to have fixed, dilated pupils.

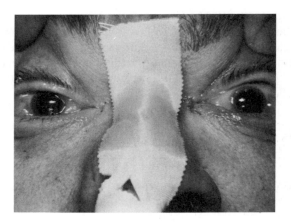

Other than mild obtundation (from sedation), results of the neuro-ophthalmic examination were normal. The patient was receiving high-dose dopamine hydrochloride for hypotension from cardiogenic shock.

Dopamine hydrochloride, when administered in high systemic doses, acts as an iris dilator. This case is an example of the toxic pupil from systemic causes. A similar picture can be seen with anticholinergic drugs, which produce a paresis of the iris sphincter.

Dilated Pupils from Uveitis

A 34-year-old woman was noted to have a fixed, dilated left pupil on routine eye examination. Ten years earlier she had developed a chronic iritis felt to be secondary to sarcoidosis. The pupil was fixed to light and accommodation, with thinning of the iris.

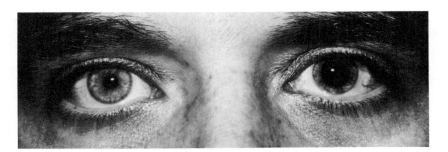

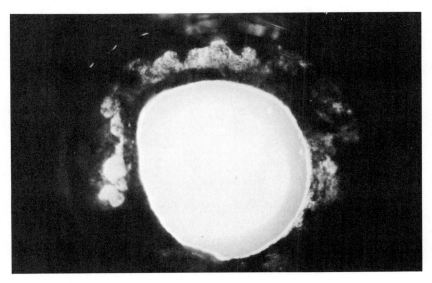

Slit lamp retroillumination

This case exemplifies iris atrophy presenting as a fixed, dilated pupil. Usually there is no difficulty on history or examination in differentiating this from the other causes of pupillary dilation.

Bibliography

Edelson, R. N., and Levy, D. E. Transient benign unilateral pupillary dilation in young adults. *Arch. Neurol.* 31:12, 1974.

Harriman, D. G. F., and Garland, H. The pathology of Adie's syndrome. *Brain* 91:401, 1968.

Loewenfeld, I. E., and Thompson, H. S. The tonic pupil: A reevaluation. *Am. J. Ophthalmol.* 63:46, 1967.

Miller, N. R., et al. Intermittent pupillary dilation in a young woman. *Surv. Ophthalmol.* 31:65, 1986.

Payne, J., and Adamkiewicz, J., Jr. Unilateral internal ophthalmoplegia with intracranial aneurysm. *Am. J. Ophthalmol.* 68:349, 1969.

Ponsford, J. R., Bannister, R., and Paul, E. A. Methacholine pupillary responses in third nerve palsy and Adie's syndrome. *Brain* 105:583, 1982.

Selhorst, J. B. The pupil and its disorders. *Neurol. Clin.* 1:859, 1983.

Thompson, H. S. Adie's syndrome: Some new observations. *Trans. Am. Ophthalmol. Soc.* 75:587, 1977.

Thompson, H. S., Newsome, D. A., and Loewenfeld, I. E. The fixed dilated pupil: Sudden iridoplegia or mydriatic drops? A simple diagnostic test. *Arch. Ophthalmol.* 86:21, 1971.

Thompson, H. S., and Pilley, S. F. J. Unequal pupils: A flow chart for sorting out the anisocorias. *Surv. Ophthalmol.* 21:45, 1976.

Woods, D., O'Connor, P. S., and Fleming, R. Episodic unilateral mydriasis and migraine. *Am. J. Ophthalmol.* 98:229, 1984.

35

Cavernous Sinus Fistula

A 57-year-old woman was evaluated for a red left eye. After multiple courses of antibiotic and steroid eyedrops, a head computed tomography (CT) scan (read as normal), and thyroid evaluations, she was referred for neuro-ophthalmic evaluation. She denied pain but did complain of blurred vision on the left and a "roaring" in her ears, which had worsened over a 6-month period. She had a history of chronic, mild hypertension.

Neuro-Ophthalmic Examination

	OD	OS
Visual acuity	20/20	20/40
Color plates correct	12 of 12	12 of 12
Pupils	Normal	Normal
Visual field	Normal	Arcuate scotomas
Fundi	Normal	Dilated retinal veins
Applanation tonometry results	17 mm Hg	27 mm Hg

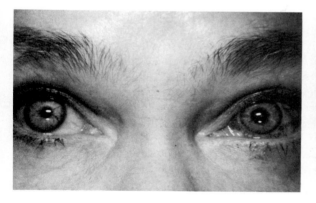 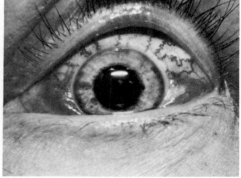

Results of a general neurologic examination were normal except for a prominent head bruit.

Summary

A middle-aged woman developed a red left eye associated with blurred vision, elevated intraocular pressure, and head bruit.

Differential Diagnosis

The evaluation of the red eye is a task that, although seemingly simple, all too frequently intimidates the best of practitioners into either unnecessary neurodiagnostic procedures or complacency in the form of the use, carte blanche, of ocular antibiotics or corticosteroids.

The external examination of the eye should give the first clue as to the presence of localized conjunctival involvement or a more extensive intraorbital process. Infection or scleral inflammation provokes a very fine conjunctival vascular response with or without concomitant exudate. The presence of dilated conjunctival veins should suggest either orbital venous obstruction or, more commonly, communication between the arterial and venous systems behind the eye (vascular malformation or fistula).

Close attention to the presence of proptosis and the pattern of the eye's redness are crucial in the differential diagnosis of this condition. Proptosis implies involvement behind the globe; retropulsion of the globe defines the degree of fullness of the orbital contents. In the patient with a full orbit from either tumor, inflammation, or blood, the globe will have resistance to retropulsion, the geography of which may indicate the type of pathology. In proptosis from a retro-orbital cause, usually venous obstruction in the cavernous sinus (from thrombosis, low flow fistula formation, or tumor mass), the globe is usually only mildly proptotic (2–4 mm) and yields easily to retropulsion.

Examination of ocular motility provides further clues as to the cause of the red eye. A restrictive motility deficit suggests intraorbital pathology. A nonrestrictive motility disturbance (cranial neuropathy) is an indication of either a posterior orbital or cavernous sinus disorder in the setting of mild proptosis. The use of forced ductions is mandatory in assessing the ocular motility disturbances in these patients. For the non-ophthalmologist this may be as simple as assessing globe movement by digitally moving the eye in the paretic direction. The optimal way to determine whether a restrictive ophthalmopathy exists is to anesthetize the eye and apply gentle traction with forceps to the muscle insertion in the direction of paretic gaze, asking the patient to look in this direction. In restrictive disorders from diffuse involvement of the muscle, such as in thyroid eye disease, the insertion may be injected, thus providing another diagnostic clue.

Last, the assessment of optic nerve function is important in the evaluation of the red eye. Optic nerve involvement implies either external compression of, or a growth within, the nerve or its coverings—such as an optic nerve glioma or nerve sheath meningioma.

In the present case, the distended conjunctival vessels suggest either venous obstruction or an increase in venous blood flow. The mild proptosis suggests a retro-orbital location for the vascular disorder. The abnormal visual acuity is easily explainable on the basis of the retinal findings, which further support the presence of a vascular disorder compromising venous drainage of the orbit. The absence of a relative afferent pupillary defect and presence of normal color vision indicate that the optic nerve is functioning normally. Elevation of the intraocular pressure is further evidence of compromise of the venous outflow system. These findings are all consistent with a fistula involving the cavernous sinus circulation. The cranial bruit is confirmatory evidence of an arteriovenous fistula.

Clinical Diagnosis: Carotid-Cavernous Sinus Fistula

The cavernous sinus is the only site within the body where a major artery passes through a venous structure. Within this intricate vascular plexus run the third, fourth, sixth, and fifth (first division) cranial nerves, as well as oculosympathetic fibers. Direct communication between the cavernous sinus and branches of the carotid artery may arise either traumatically or spontaneously.

The arteriovenous shunting present in carotid-cavernous fistulae leads to orbital venous congestion and a secondary restrictive ophthalmopathy because of boggy extraocular muscles. These same vascular dynamics within the cavernous sinus may lead to ischemia of the cranial nerves. Thus, the ocular motility in patients with carotid-cavernous fistula may be abnormal through a combination of primary muscle involvement and cranial nerve compromise. The elevated intraocular pressure is due to an increase in episcleral venous pressure, which produces a decrease in aqueous outflow. Resulting retinal ischemia and secondary glaucoma may combine to compromise visual function (Table 35-1).

Spontaneous fistulae are usually the result of dural shunts between branch arteries of the internal or external carotid and the cavernous sinus. These shunts are seen more commonly in middle-aged women than in other groups, involve the left eye more often than the right, and may be extremely difficult to identify in mild cases. Patients with this type of fistula typically present with a red eye and may or may not have a sensation of noise (bruit) behind the eye. These symptoms may be accompanied by a variable amount of pain, diplopia, and proptosis. Infrequently, these patients may have an ocular motility disturbance, usually a sixth nerve paresis, for months before the red eye and proptosis become apparent.

Table 35-1. Complications of carotid-cavernous fistula

1. Glaucomatous optic nerve damage
2. Epithelial edema, keratopathy
3. Uveitis
4. Late development of cataract
5. Dilated retinal veins
   a. Retinal hemorrhages, exudates
   b. Microaneurysms
   c. Chronic hypoxic retinopathy
6. Ocular motility disturbance
7. Iatrogenic trauma (from overexuberant treatment)

Table 35-2. Radiologic features of carotid-cavernous fistula

1. Normal computed tomography scan or
   a. Distended superior ophthalmic vein
   b. Proptosis
   c. Thickened extraocular muscles (especially medial rectus)
   d. "Bowing" of the cavernous sinus region of enhancement on contrast study
2. Arteriographic appearance depends on the arterial supply; the two most common contributing arteries in the spontaneous variety are
   a. Internal maxillary artery (external carotid)
   b. Meningohypophyseal trunk (internal carotid)

Additional Testing

The neuroimaging features of carotid-cavernous fistula are listed in Table 35-2. In a traumatic carotid-cavernous fistula, the communication between artery and vein is usually extensive, resulting in prominent orbital venous distention, which may be seen on CT scan as a dilated superior ophthalmic vein and occasionally as large, edematous muscles. Cerebral angiography confirms the presence of the fistula, and when selective injections are carried out using either conventional or digital subtraction (arterial) techniques, the source of the fistula may be visualized.

In the spontaneous variety of dural shunt fistula, the CT scan findings may be the same but are often more subtle. Cerebral angiography using selective catheterization is necessary to identify the specific internal or external carotid artery branch responsible for the dural shunt. The procedure of cerebral angiography itself may be enough to close off the fistula in the spontaneous variety.

In patients with traumatic fistula between the cavernous sinus and internal carotid artery, cerebral angiography is necessary in all cases to plan the appropriate treatment. In the spontaneous variety of dural shunt fistula, a CT scan of the cavernous sinus and orbits may be sufficient to confirm the diagnosis. We obtain intraarterial digital subtraction angiography (with selective catheterization) only in symptomatic patients to identify the arterial branches responsible for the fistula. If fistula closure then becomes necessary, a rational approach to selective catheterization can be planned in advance.

Treatment

The treatment of carotid-cavernous fistula depends on the severity of the arteriovenous shunt and the secondary effect of the fistula on the orbital contents. The rationale for any of the various treatments in carotid-cavernous fistula is based on closing the arteriovenous shunt. Historically this closure was done by tying off the ipsilateral internal carotid artery. The difficulty with occluding the carotid is that other intracranial structures are then at risk for ischemia. In addition, the goal of the treatment, that is, visual preservation through reduction of orbital ischemia, is further compromised with more ischemia produced by a further reduction in arterial flow owing to the carotid ligation. Because of the

Table 35-3. Evaluation and management of carotid-cavernous fistula

1. Baseline external and fundus photos
2. Assessment of optic nerve function
3. Evaluation of visual fields
4. Intraocular pressure determination
5. Arteriography, computed tomography scan, digital intraarterial studies
   a. If there is any question of the diagnosis
   b. In trauma patients
   c. If treatment with interventional techniques is being considered
6. Reassurance and close follow-up of visual function in minimally symptomatic cases of dural fistulae

complications of carotid ligation, selective catheterization of the offending artery with the introduction of glue, balloons, or plastic spheres to close off the arterial rent have recently been pioneered in interventional radiology. The type of treatment selected depends on the type of fistula, degree of patient compromise, and skill of the interventional radiologist available.

The treatment of spontaneous carotid-cavernous fistula and treatment of the traumatic type are best discussed separately.

Spontaneous Dural Fistula
Occasionally, the spontaneous variety of dural shunt fistula resolves spontaneously. Some fistulae even resolve during the angiographic procedures used to evaluate them. Since the various methods of treating these fistulae may lead to morbidity (and even mortality) not seen in the natural history of the untreated disease, a conservative approach is advisable. If there is little or no visual function compromise and the patient can tolerate the symptoms, such fistulae are best left untreated except for intraocular pressure reduction. In untreated patients it is important to follow visual function along with the patient's symptoms (Table 35-3); if there is a sudden worsening of the clinical picture, then interventional radiology is indicated to attempt closing off the fistula.

Traumatic Carotid-Cavernous Fistula
In the traumatic fistula, the rent in the carotid artery will not close spontaneously, and the degree of orbital vascular compromise or patient discomfort is usually sufficient to warrant the risks of treatment. In these patients we opt for an interventional radiologic approach, using the balloon technique. If this is ineffective, then the artery is ligated gradually, with the patient observed (in the hospital) for symptoms of cerebral ischemia.

Management and Course of the Case
CT scan of the head demonstrated prominent extraocular muscle thickening with distention of the superior ophthalmic vein and outward bowing of the cavernous sinus.

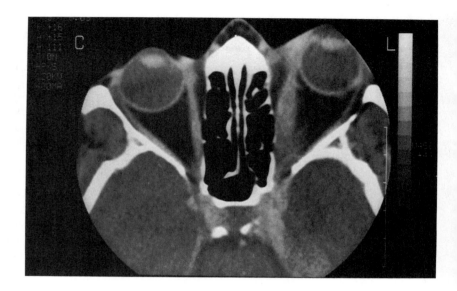

Arteriography demonstrated a meningohypophyseal dural fistula.

The patient was treated with timolol maleate (Timoptic) eyedrops to reduce her intraocular pressure. Over a period of 16 months she had gradual resolution of the proptosis, with persistence of mildly dilated conjunctival vessels and a visual acuity of 20/40 on the involved side.

Traumatic Carotid-Cavernous Fistula

A 40-year-old woman was noted to have marked orbital edema and proptosis after a closed head injury. Visual acuity was 20/100 with impaired color vision and an ischemic retina on funduscopy. Ocular motility tests showed almost a complete ophthalmoplegia with some restrictive component. CT scan demonstrated a markedly enlarged superior ophthalmic vein (see p. 251).

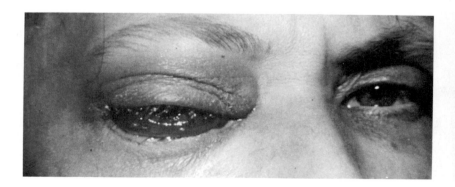

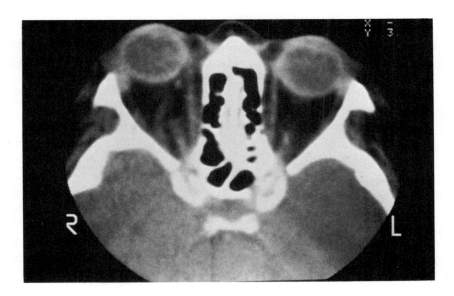

This case is a typical presentation of a traumatic carotid-cavernous fistula with secondary retinal ischemia and ocular motility disturbance.

Traumatic carotid-cavernous fistulae usually follow major head injuries. These fistulae do not regress spontaneously and are often associated with serious visual morbidity. The treatment, as outlined in the foregoing case, consists of attempting to close the rent in the carotid artery as it traverses the cavernous sinus. The advent of interventional radiology, with its refinement of intraarterial glue and balloon placements (in specific arterial distributions), has revolutionized the treatment of central nervous system vascular disorders. This type of treatment should only be carried out, however, by an interventionist well versed (and well practiced) in the techniques available.

Glaucoma from Cavernous Sinus Fistula

A 45-year-old man had been followed for a red eye and glaucoma for 4 years. Visual acuity was 20/20 in each eye with pressures of 32 mm Hg in the right eye and 14 mm Hg in the left and marked cupping of the right disk. There was diffuse dilation of the conjunctival veins of the right eye. A clinical diagnosis of arteriovenous cavernous sinus fistula was made. Angiography was not performed as the diagnosis was firm clinically. Trabeculectomy was performed rather than consideration for shunt closure.

Bibliography

Bickerstaff, E. R. Mechanisms of presentation of caroticocavernous fistulae. *Br. J. Ophthalmol.* 54:186, 1970.

Debrun, G., et al. Treatment of 54 traumatic carotid-cavernous fistulas. *J. Neurosurg.* 55:678, 1981.

Fleishman, J. A., Garfinkle, R. A., and Beck, R. W. Advances in the treatment of carotid-cavernous fistulas. *Int. Ophthalmol. Clin.* 26 (4): 301, 1986.

Grove, A. S. The dural shunt syndrome: Pathophysiology and clinical course. *Ophthalmology* 91:31, 1984.

Harris, F. S., and Rhoton, A. L. Anatomy of the cavernous sinus: A microsurgical study. *J. Neurosurg.* 45:169, 1976.

Newton, T. H., and Hoyt, W. F. Dural arteriovenous shunts in the region of the cavernous sinus. *Neuroradiology* 1:71, 1970.

Nukui, H., et al. Long-term observations in cases with spontaneous carotid-cavernous fistulas. *Surg. Neurol.* 21:543, 1984.

Parkinson, D. Collateral circulation of cavernous carotid artery: Anatomy. *Can. J. Surg.* 7:251, 1964.

Parkinson, D. Carotid-Cavernous Fistula: Direct Approach and Repair of Fistula and Preservation of the Artery. In T. P. Morley, *Current Controversies in Neurosurgery.* Philadelphia: Saunders, 1976.

Phelps, C. D., Thompson, H. S., and Ossonig, K. C. The diagnosis and prognosis of atypical carotid-cavernous fistula (red-eyed shunt syndrome). *Am. J. Ophthalmol.* 93:423, 1982.

Saunders, M. D., and Hoyt, W. F. Hypoxic ocular sequelae of carotid-cavernous fistulae: Study of the causes of visual failure before and after neurosurgical treatment in a series of 25 cases. *Br. J. Ophthalmol.* 53:82, 1969.

West, C. S. H. Bilateral carotid-cavernous fistulae: A review. *Surg. Neurol.* 13:85, 1980.

36

Essential Blepharospasm

A 63-year-old woman had an insidious worsening of eyelid spasms over the 3-year period before examination. She noted that the spasms would worsen in stressful situations and toward the end of the day. She had been treated with numerous antianxiety and psychotropic medications without improvement and had contemplated suicide since becoming unable to work or interact socially because of continual eyelid closure.

Neuro-Ophthalmic Examination

	OU
Visual acuity	20/20
Color plates correct	10 of 10
Pupils	Normal
Visual field	Normal (with taped eyelids)
Fundi	Normal
Lids	Bilateral asynchronous eyelid spasms

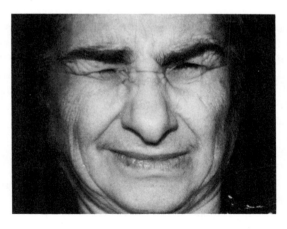

A general neurologic examination revealed minimal oral and facial dystonic movements.

Summary
A 63-year-old woman had slowly progressive bilateral orbicularis oculi and facial spasms.

Table 36-1. Types of eyelid spasm

Localization	Unilateral	Bilateral
Supranuclear	Focal seizures	Essential blepharospasm Meige's disease
Nuclear	Myokymia	—
Infranuclear	Hemifacial spasm Synkinetic movements	—
Other	—	Reflex blepharospasm Habit spasm (tic)

Differential Diagnosis

Facial movement disorders can be broadly grouped according to whether facial involvement is unilateral or bilateral. These movements can be further classified into disorders of supranuclear, nuclear, or infranuclear facial nerve (Table 36-1). When bilateral, orbicularis spasms are due to essential blepharospasm, habit spasm (tic), or reflex blepharospasm. The differential of unilateral eyelid spasms is more extensive and is reviewed in the next case.

Reflex blepharospasm is caused by either anterior segment ocular inflammation or referred trigeminal nerve pain from retro-orbital or meningeal disease. Patients with reflex blepharospasm usually have control over their spasms and often complain of photophobia, a symptom not encountered in the other types of eyelid spasm and facial movement disorders. These patients prefer to keep their eyes closed, whereas in habit spasm and essential blepharospasm, the patients' primary complaint is eyelid closure.

Habit spasm is a stereotyped complex facial movement created volitionally and easily suppressed. Patients with habit spasm are generally not inconvenienced by the movements, which lessen in intensity when not socially observed.

This patient's bilateral eyelid spasms were involuntary, not associated with external eye or meningeal disease, and associated with a more general facial movement disorder. Essential blepharospasm is the most likely diagnosis.

Clinical Diagnosis: Essential Blepharospasm

In a majority of patients, an orbicularis oculi spasm will be found to fall under the rubric of essential blepharospasm. This is a disorder that has mystified clinicians for over a century; frequently misdiagnosed, it more often than not defies treatment even when correctly identified.

Essential blepharospasm generally has its onset between the ages of 45 and 60 years; excessive blinking is the usual first symptom. This blinking gradually intensifies, insidiously becoming a spasm of the eyelid that is not under volitional control. Although involvement may be unilateral early in the course of the disease, it eventually becomes bilateral, producing impairment of visual function that limits activities of daily life. With progression of the disease, approximately 12 percent of patients become functionally blind, and many withdraw from all social contact.

Most patients find that their symptoms are relieved with sleep or rest and that the spasms are absent or markedly less severe in the morning and at their worst in the afternoon. Activities involving conversation or other social intercourse or emotional stress frequently precipitate uncontrollable spasms—a factor leading to further social withdrawal.

When it is entirely unilateral (an unusual occurrence), essential blepharospasm is frequently confused with habit spasm (facial tic) or, occasionally, with hemifacial spasm (see below). The majority of patients, however, when observed closely, will be seen to have bilateral involvement; thus, unnecessary diagnostic procedures and treatments can be avoided. Careful clinical observation will also reveal other signs of abnormal movements of the lower facial musculature and neck, and in a large percentage of patients there will be frank signs of basal ganglion dysfunction.

When blepharospasm is seen in association with mouth retraction, facial grimacing, jaw opening, and retrocollic spasms, the clinical features suggest more widespread basal ganglion dysfunction than seen in essential blepharospasm. Described initially by Meige in 1910, the more widespread disease presents initially as essential blepharospasm; the additional movements appear insidiously over many years. This entity has been variably referred to as Meige's disease, blepharospasm-oromandibular dystonia, and idiopathic orofacial dystonia. The exact distinction between these entities and essential blepharospasm with additional dystonic posturings has not been clearly defined.

Additional Testing
Once a diagnosis of essential blepharospasm is made clinically, no further testing need be done.

Treatment
The overall appearance of patients with essential blepharospasm and Meige's disease, with their bizarre posturings, has prompted many clinicians to treat them as if they had an underlying psychiatric disorder. Consequently, a variety of antipsychotic, antidepressant, and muscle-relaxant medications have been tried—with little success. These medications may lead to a tardive dyskinesia that is difficult to differentiate from the dystonic posturings seen in Meige's disease, further confusing the clinical picture.

Two therapies are beneficial in essential blepharospasm: orbicularis stripping and botulinum (Oculinum) injections. The former is a laborious surgical procedure that usually controls the symptoms in about 80 percent of patients. Oculinum injections provide a novel, well-tolerated approach in which botulinum toxin is injected into the orbicularis oculi musculature, providing temporary relief of the spasms for up to 3 or

4 months. The latter procedure can be performed on an outpatient basis with a minimum of morbidity.

Patients who have blepharospasm with or without accompanying orofacial dystonia may be profoundly depressed, whether as a result of the underlying disease or secondary to the incapacitating facial movements. Management of these cases should include close psychiatric observation, particularly during therapeutic trials of potentially toxic medications with the potential for being abused.

Management and Course of the Case

The patient underwent a series of Oculinum injections, which provided excellent control of the eyelid spasms and allowed a return to functional status. Her depression cleared. A majority of her other facial dystonic movements improved, although these muscle groups were not directly affected by the botulinum toxin injections.

Hemifacial Spasm

A 52-year-old man noted the onset of left eyelid twitching, which insidiously worsened over a 3-year period to involve the entire left side of his face. He denied other neurologic symptoms with the exception of a clicking noise in his right ear when the spasm was at its peak. Rhythmic, intermittent facial twitching was noted to involve the entire left side of the patient's face, including the platysma musculature. Findings of the remainder of the neuro-ophthalmic examination were normal.

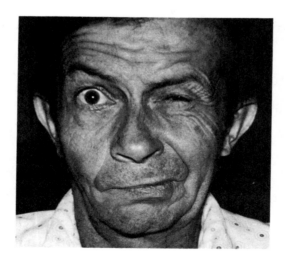

Unilateral eyelid spasms and facial twitching can be a manifestation of focal cortical seizures, synkinetic movements, or hemifacial spasm.

1. *Synkinetic movements.* Axonal compression or disruption at any point along the course of the facial nerve may lead either to aberrant regeneration or to ephaptic transmission in adjacent axons. *Aberrant regeneration* refers to the resprouting of axons down incorrect myelin sheaths after disruption of the nerve. *Ephaptic transmission* refers to the concept of an "artificial synapse" between contiguous nerves, created by a disruption of the normally directed electrical or chemical transmission along a single nerve trunk. Whatever the mechanism, this misdirected neural firing leads to the synchronous firing of unassociated muscle groups in response to minor voluntary contractions. The resulting movements (synkinesias) become apparent within weeks to months after the neural insult and may progress to the point of spastic hemifacial contracture. The usual appearance clinically is that of orbicularis oris contraction (cheek puckering) with minimal eyelid closure.

2. *Focal cortical seizures.* Rarely, epileptiform discharges arising from a localized cortical region will be manifested by gross clonic movements involving one side of the face. These movements, when closely inspected, are seen to involve contiguous cortical areas, manifested by motor activity beyond the distribution of the facial nerve. Postictally there is usually a supranuclear type of paresis (e.g., Todd's paresis), which represents exhaustion of the cortical tonic input. These patients should be considered to have focal cortical disease and prompt neuroanatomic studies should be carried out to direct the appropriate treatment course.

3. *Hemifacial spasm.* Rhythmic, intermittent, unilateral facial twitching, which begins insidiously around the orbicularis oculi and spreads slowly over a period of 1 to 5 years to involve all of the muscles of facial expression, is characteristic of hemifacial spasm. These bursts of tonic (or clonic) activity may last only seconds or may continue for minutes to hours. They are exacerbated by stressful situations and may occur during sleep. They may intensify for days, then subside and abate for weeks to months—only to recur in a relentless progression. This movement disorder tends to affect women more frequently than men, and the left side of the face is more often involved than the right. Typically after courses of muscle relaxants, antidepressants, and psychotherapy, the disease becomes prominent enough to be recognized as not being of psychogenic origin.

In this patient the history and findings are most consistent with hemifacial spasm.

Although occasionally patients give a history of antecedent ipsilateral facial palsy and therefore have their condition called *postparalytic* hemifacial spasm, most do not, and their disease falls under the rubric of *cryptogenic* hemifacial spasm.

Gardner and Sava postulated that damage from compression or other injury to the facial nerve in its extraaxial course produces increased irritability with spontaneous firing in hemifacial spasm. The concept of a spread of impulses between axons of the nerves (ephaptic transmission) has been set forth to explain how fibers directed toward one muscle group might excite adjacent nerve fibers directed to another muscle group. This ephaptic transmission, if present, probably occurs in the root exit zone in the cerebellopontine angle. Although both extraaxial and intraaxial lesions have been described in association with hemifacial spasm, it is believed that in the majority of patients nerve compression is caused by a tortuous anterior or posterior inferior cerebellar artery.

The prolonged, severe contractions of facial musculature lead to an annoying, and frequently cosmetically disfiguring, grimacing with partial eyelid closure. Although this grimacing is usually painless, patients may complain of mouth or neck pains with severe contractions and of an occasional sensation of oscillopsia and auditory sensations from lid and tensor tympani spasm.

Although carbamazepine (Tegretol) has provided transient relief in some patients, the disease tends to be relentless in progression and unresponsive to medical therapy.

Patients with the cryptogenic form of hemifacial spasm have impressive improvement after suboccipital craniotomy with placement of a cushion between the offending vessel and nerve. Although Janetta and colleagues have found this procedure to be curative in over 90 percent of patients, the morbidity is not negligible: hearing loss ipsilaterally (8%), facial paralysis (4%), and posterior fossa subdural hematomas (rare) have been reported as complications.

Oculinum injections have also proved beneficial in hemifacial spasm, particularly when the majority of the movement disorder is localized to the orbicularis oculi region.

In cases of mild hemifacial spasm, after appropriate neuroimaging modalities have demonstrated no tumor, the prudent course is to reassure the patient and follow without treatment. When the spasms become socially unacceptable, Oculinum injections, if available, provide palliation. If the definitive posterior fossa craniotomy is to be utilized, the patient should be willing to accept the possible risks of the procedure.

Facial Myokymia

A 30-year-old woman noted right facial "movements" that came on concomitantly with diplopia on left gaze. Three years previously she had noted blurred vision in her left eye for a period of 2 weeks associated with mild pain on eye movement. Neuro-ophthalmic examination showed a left relative afferent pupillary defect, normal visual acuity, and nerve fiber layer loss in both eyes on funduscopy. Ocular motility testing showed a subclinical right internuclear ophthalmoplegia.

This patient has right facial myokymia. The examination localized the lesion to the region of the right pons. The bilateral optic nerve disease indicates multiple lesions in space (and over time, by history), strongly suggesting the diagnosis of demyelinating disease (multiple sclerosis).

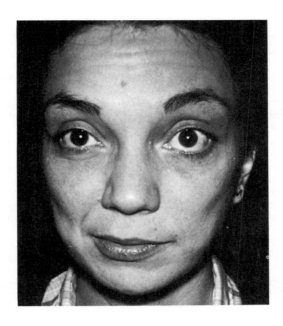

When nuclear lesions increase lower motor neuron activity, the facial muscles contract in a continual, undulating, involuntary manner, involving predominantly the periocular and orbicularis oris musculature. This type of vermiform movement disorder of the face is called facial myokymia and signifies intramedullary disease of the pons involving the facial nucleus or fascicle. Although infrequently seen in the Guillain-Barré syndrome, it is virtually pathognomonic for either a pontine glioma (in patients younger than 10 years of age) or demyelinating disease (in patients older than 15 years). Brainstem tuberculoma also has been reported to cause facial myokymia. This movement disorder is perceived by the patient as a "nervous twitch" and rarely arises unaccompanied by other neurologic signs or symptoms. Facial myokymia should be differentiated from the normal transient twitches of extreme fatigue and from the rhythmic contractions seen in hemifacial spasm.

Treatment of this movement disorder should be aimed at the underlying pathology. If the underlying disease cannot be treated and the myokymic movements are socially unacceptable, carbamazepine (Tegretol) or phenytoin (Dilantin) may be of benefit.

Bibliography

Andermann, F., et al. Facial myokymia in multiple sclerosis. *Brain* 81:31, 1961.

Ehni, G., and Woltman, H. W. Hemifacial spasm: Review of one hundred and six cases. *Arch. Neurol. Psychiatry* 53:205, 1945.

Frueh, B. R., et al. Treatment of blepharospasm with botulinum toxin. *Arch. Ophthalmol.* 102:1464, 1984.

Gardner, W. J., and Sava, G. A. Hemifacial spasm: A reversible pathophysiologic state. *J. Neurosurg.* 19:240, 1962.

Gillum, W. N., and Anderson, R. L. Blepharospasm surgery: An anatomical approach. *Arch. Ophthalmol.* 99:1056, 1981.

Henderson, J. W. Essential blepharospasm. *Trans. Am. Ophthalmol. Soc.* 54:453, 1956.

Jankovic, J., Havins, W. E., and Wilkins, R. B. Blinking and blepharospasm. *J.A.M.A.* 248:3160, 1982.

Jannetta, P. J., et al. Etiology and definitive microsurgical treatment of hemifacial spasm: Operative techniques and results in 47 patients. *J. Neurosurg.* 47:321, 1977.

Loeser, J. D., and Chen, J. Hemifacial spasm: Treatment by microsurgical facial nerve decompression. *Neurosurgery* 13:141, 1983.

Marsden, C. D. Blepharospasm—oromandibular dystonia syndrome (Brueghel's syndrome): A variant of adult onset torsion dystonia? *J. Neurol. Neurosurg. Psychiatry* 39:1204, 1976.

McCord, C. D., et al. Treatment of essential blepharospasm: I. Comparison of facial nerve avulsion and eyebrow-eyelid muscle stripping procedure. *Arch. Ophthalmol.* 102:266, 1984.

McCord, C. D., Shore, J., and Putnam, J. R. Treatment of essential blepharospasm: II. A modification of exposure for the muscle stripping technique. *Arch. Ophthalmol.* 102:269, 1984.

Miller, N. M., et al. "Squeezing eyes": A clinicopathologic conference. *Surv. Ophthalmol.* 26:97, 1981.

Nielsen, V. K., and Jannetta, P. J. Pathophysiology of hemifacial spasm: III. Effects of facial nerve decompression. *Neurology* 34:891, 1984.

Perman, K. I., et al. The use of botulinum toxin in the medical management of benign essential blepharospasm. *Ophthalmology* 93:1, 1986.

Piatt, J. H., and Wilkins, R. H. Treatment of tic douloureux and hemifacial spasm by posterior fossa exploration: Therapeutic implications of various neurovascular relationships. *Neurosurgery* 14:462, 1984.

Renser, R. B., and Corbett, J. J. Myokymia and facial contraction in brainstem glioma. *Arch. Neurol.* 30:425, 1974.

Savino, P. J., et al. Hemifacial spasm treated with botulinum A toxin injection. *Arch Ophthalmol.* 103:1305, 1985.

Scott, A. B., Kennedy, R. A., and Stubbs, H. A. Botulinum A toxin injection as a treatment for blepharospasm. *Arch. Ophthalmol.* 103:347, 1985.

Shorr, N., Seiff, S. R., and Kopelman, J. The use of botulinum toxin in blepharospasm. *Am. J. Ophthalmol.* 99:542, 1985.

Smith, C. H., and Beck, R. W. Facial Nerve. In T. D. Duane and E. A. Jaeger (eds.), *Biomedical Foundations of Ophthalmology.* Philadelphia: Harper & Row, 1983.

Tsoy, E. A., Buckley, E. G., and Dutton, J. J. Treatment of blepharospasm with botulinum toxin. *Am. J. Ophthalmol.* 99:176, 1985.

Wartenberg, R. *Hemifacial Spasm: A Clinical and Pathophysiological Study.* New York; London: Oxford University Press, 1952.

Waybright, E. A., Gutman, L., and Chou, S. M. Facial myokymia: Pathological features. *Arch. Neurol.* 36:244, 1979.

Index

Abducens nerve. *See* Sixth nerve palsy.
Abduction deficit, differential diagnosis of, 28, 189
Aberrant regeneration
  after facial nerve palsy, 257
  after third nerve palsy, 170–171, 174–175
Acetylcholine receptor antibody titer, in myasthenia gravis, 224
Achromatopsia, congenital, 104
Adduction deficits. *See also* Internuclear ophthalmoplegia.
  differential diagnosis of, 198–199
  in myasthenia gravis, 203–204
Adie's pupil, 239–241
Albinism, 104–105
Alternating light test, 4–7
Amaurosis, Leber's congenital, 104
Amaurosis fugax, 106–110
  in young adult, 108–109
Amblyopia, tobacco-alcohol, 93
Amsler grid, 9
Aneurysm
  cavernous sinus, 176–177
  causing third nerve palsy, 172
Anisocoria. *See also* Pupil, dilated.
  evaluation of, 31–33
Anterior ischemic optic neuropathy, 46–51
  arteritic, with normal sedimentation rate in, 50–51
  arteritic vs nonarteritic, 47
  bilateral, giant cell arteritis and, 56–57
  differential diagnosis of, 47
  giant cell arteritis and, 54–55
  optic disk drusen and, 70
Arteriovenous malformation, 146–147

Bielschowsky three-step test, 28–30
Blepharospasm, essential, 253–256
Blepharospasm-oromandibular dystonia, 255
Blowout fracture, 160
Bromocriptine mesylate, 124

Carotid-cavernous fistula, 245–252
  glaucoma from, 251
  spontaneous dural, 249
  traumatic, 249, 250–251
Carotid artery disease, amaurosis fugax in, 107
Cavernous sinus
  aneurysm, 176–177
  fistula, 245–252
  meningioma, 158–159

Chiasmal syndrome. *See* Optic chiasm.
Color vision, evaluation of, 2
Compressive optic neuropathy, 73–79
  thyroid, 114–115
Cone dystrophy, 94–95
Convergence spasm, 194–196
Cortical blindness, 140–141
  in infant, 104
Cortical seizure, focal, 257
Craniopharyngioma, 132–134
  as optic neuritis mimic, 39–40

Diabetes mellitus
  juvenile, recessive optic atrophy in, 87
  papillopathy in, 113
Diplopia
  causes of, 27–30
  evaluation of, 26–30
Dopamine hydrochloride, dilated pupils due to, 242–243
Dorsal midbrain syndrome, 179–183
Downgaze, limitation of, 28
Drusen, optic disk. *See also* Pseudopapilledema.
  anterior ischemic optic neuropathy and, 70
  pituitary tumor and, 69
  progressive visual loss in, 70–72
Duane's retraction syndrome, 193–194

Electromyogram, single-fiber, 224
Endarterectomy, 107
Esotropia, causes of, 28
Exotropia, causes of, 27–28
Eyelid spasm, types of, 254

Facial myokymia, 258–259
Facial nerve, aberrant regeneration of, 257
Fisher's syndrome, 205–208
Fourth nerve palsy, 163–167
  congenital, 166–167
  three-step test in, 30
Foville's syndrome, 190
Functional visual loss, 148–152

Geniculocalcarine visual system, lesions of, 23–26
Giant cell arteritis, 53–57
  in anterior ischemic optic neuropathy, 54–55
  with bilateral anterior ischemic optic neuropathy, 56–57
  with normal sedimentation rate, 50–51
  temporal artery biopsy in, 55

Glaucoma
    binasal defects from, 130
    from cavernous sinus fistula, 251
Glioma
    optic chiasm, 81
    optic nerve, 80–83
Graves' ophthalmopathy, 153–158
    abduction deficit in, 192–193
    limited upgaze in, 153–158
    optic neuropathy, 114–115
Guillain-Barré syndrome. See Fisher's
    syndrome.

Hemifacial spasm, 256–258
Heterophoria, 27
Hollenhorst plaque, 109
Homonymous hemianopia, 23–26,
    136–143
    from occipital lobe lesion, 137–139
    from parietal lobe lesion, 141–142
    from temporal lobe lesions, 142–143
Horner's syndrome, 33, 230, 234–238
    in child, 238
Hypertension, malignant, optic disk edema
    in, 65
Hysterical blindness. See Functional visual
    loss.

Infant
    albinism in, 104–105
    congenital achromatopsia in, 104
    cortical blindness in, 104
    developmental delay in, 103–104
    Leber's congenital amaurosis in, 104
    with poor vision, differential diagnosis
        in, 103–105
    retinal disorders in, 104–105
    visual evaluation in, 2
Internuclear ophthalmoplegia, 197–204
    bilateral, 201–203
    walleyed bilateral, 202–203
Ischemic optic neuropathy. See Anterior is-
    chemic optic neuropathy.

Kearns-Sayre syndrome, 208–210
Koerber-Salus-Elschnig syndrome, 180

Lateral rectus palsy. See Sixth nerve palsy.
Leber's congenital amaurosis, 104
Leber's optic neuropathy, 88–91
Leber's stellate maculopathy, 44
Lid retraction, 232–233
Light brightness comparison test, 19

Macular disease, optic nerve disorders vs,
    19
Macular sparing, definition of, 8
Malingering. See Functional visual loss.
Marcus-Gunn test, 4–6
Meige's disease, 255
Meningioma
    bilateral central scotoma in, 95–97
    compressive optic neuropathy and,
        74–76

junctional scotoma from, 77
    optic nerve sheath, 74–75
    optociliary shunt vessels from, 78
    sphenoid wing, 74–75, 158–159
    tuberculum sellae or planum
        sphenoidale, 74–75
Meningitis, ophthalmoplegia from,
    212–213
Migraine, 144–147
    acephalgic, 145
    arteriovenous malformation mimicking,
        146–147
    transient visual loss due to, 108–109
Möbius' syndrome, 213–214
Mucocele, sphenoidal, 38
Multiple sclerosis
    internuclear ophthalmoplegia, 197–202
    optic neuritis and, 35, 37
Muscular dystrophy, oculopharyngeal, 210
Myasthenia gravis, 221–227
    acetylcholine receptor antibody titer in,
        224
    adduction deficit from, 203–204
    curariform drug tests in, 224–225
    limited upgaze in, 161
    neostigmine bromide (Prostigmin) test,
        224
    pseudo-lid retraction in, 233
    ptosis in, 226–227
    repetitive nerve stimulation in, 224
    single-fiber electromyogram in, 224
    Tensilon test in, 223–224
Myokymia, facial, 258–259

Neostigmine bromide (Prostigmin) test, in
    myasthenia gravis, 224
Neuro-ophthalmic examination, 1–33
    oculomotor system evaluation in,
        26–33
    visual function evaluation in, 1–24
Neurofibromatosis, optic glioma in, 80–82
Neuroretinitis, 44
Nutritional optic neuropathy, 92–97
Nystagmus
    congenital, 31
    evaluation of, 30–31
    types of, neurologic localization of, 31

Occipital lobe lesion
    cortical blindness from, 140–141
    homonymous hemianopia from,
        136–140
    localization of, 14
Oculomotor nerve palsy. See Third nerve
    palsy.
Oculomotor system, evaluation of, 26–30
Oculopharyngeal muscular dystrophy,
    210–211
Oculosympathetic paresis, 230, 234–238.
    See also Horner's syndrome.
Ophthalmoplegia
    chronic progressive external, 208–210
    internuclear, 197–204. See also Inter-
        nuclear ophthalmoplegia.

from meningitis, 212–213
Optic atrophy, differential diagnosis, 20
Optic atrophy, hereditary, 84–87. *See also* Leber's optic neuropathy.
  dominant, 84–86
  recessive with juvenile diabetes, 87
Optic chiasm, 122–131
  anatomy, 20
  demyelination of, 127–128
  differential diagnosis, 20–23
  glioma of, 80–83
  localization of lesions of, 14
  pituitary tumor affecting, 122–127
  traumatic injury to, 100
Optic disk
  in optic nerve disorders, 16–20
    atrophy of, 20
    edema of, 16–18. *See also* Papilledema.
    normal, 19–20
  tilted, 129
Optic disk drusen
  anterior ischemic optic neuropathy and, 70
  pituitary tumor and, 69
  progressive visual loss in, 70–72
  in pseudopapilledema. *See* Pseudopapilledema.
Optic disk infarct, 116
Optic nerve disorders, 14–20
  central scotoma in, 14–16
  macular disease vs, 19
  nerve fiber bundle defects in, 16
  optic disk appearance in, 16–20
  time course of visual loss in, 18
  visual field defects in, 14–16
Optic nerve glioma, 80–83
  neurofibromatosis and, 80–82
Optic nerve hypoplasia, 102–105
Optic nerve sheath
  decompression of, in pseudotumor cerebri, 62–63
  meningioma of, 74–75
Optic neuritis, 34–41
  in child, 42–44
  multiple sclerosis and, 35, 37
Optic neuropathy
  anterior ischemic, 46–51. *See also* Anterior ischemic optic neuropathy.
  compressive, 73–79
  diabetic, 113
  differential diagnosis of, 14–20
  Leber's, 88–91
  nutritional, 92–97
  radiation, 119
  retrobulbar ischemic, 55
  sarcoid, 115–116
  shock, 117
  syphilitic, 118
  thyroid, 114–115
  traumatic, 98–101
Optic tract syndrome, 14, 23, 132–133
  demyelination, 134–135

Optociliary shunt vessels, from meningioma, 78
Orbital apex syndrome, 216–218
Orbital fracture, 160
Orofacial dystonia, idiopathic, 255

Papilledema
  early, pseudopapilledema vs, 67
  funduscopic changes in, 60
  in increased intracranial pressure, 18, 59–60
Papillitis, 38
Papillopathy, in diabetes mellitus, 113
Papillophlebitis, 111
Parasympathetic pupillary pathway, anatomy of, 32
Parietal lobe lesion
  homonymous hemianopia from, 23–24, 141–142
  localization of, 14
Parinaud's syndrome. *See* Dorsal midbrain syndrome.
Photostress test, 19
Pilocarpine test, in dilated pupil, 31, 240
Pituitary tumor, 122–124
  apoplexy, 125–127
  clinical diagnosis of, 123–124
  optic disk drusen and, 69
Pretectal syndrome. *See* Dorsal midbrain syndrome.
Prism shift test, 152
Prostigmin test, in myasthenia gravis, 224
Pseudo-Foster Kennedy syndrome, 49–50
Pseudo-lid retraction, in myasthenia, 233
Pseudo-von Graefe phenomenon, 170
Pseudodrusen, in papilledema, 60
Pseudopapilledema, 66–72
  early papilledema vs, 67
Pseudotumor cerebri, 58–65
  diplopia in, 60
  lumbar puncture in, 60–61
  optic nerve sheath decompression in, 62–63
  progressive visual loss in, 62–64
Ptosis
  bilateral, from brainstem lesion, 229
  congenital, 228
  in Horner's syndrome, 230, 234–238
  in myasthenia gravis, 226–227
  senile, 227
Pupil
  afferent pupillary defect, 4–7
  dilated, 33, 239–244
    in Adie's (tonic pupil) syndrome, 239–241
    from dopamine hydrochloride, 242–243
    pharmacologic, 241–242
    pilocarpine test in, 240
    in uveitis, 243
  evaluation of, 2–7, 31–33
  Horner's syndrome, 234–238
  pharmacologic testing, 31
  tonic, 239–241

Radiation optic neuropathy, 119
Red eye, evaluation of, 246–247
Repetitive nerve stimulation, in myasthenia gravis, 224
Retinal disorders, in infant, 104–105
Retinal nerve fibers, distribution of, at optic nerve, 16
Retinal vein, central, partial occlusion of, 112
Retrobulbar ischemic optic neuropathy, 55
Retrobulbar neuritis, 38

Sarcoid optic neuropathy, 115–116
Scotoma
    bilateral central, 16
        causes of, 93
        from meningioma, 95–97
    definition of, 8
    junctional, from meningioma, 77
    scintillating, 137
    unilateral central, 14–16
Seizure, focal cortical, 257
Septo-optic dysplasia syndrome, 103
Shock optic neuropathy, 117
Sixth nerve palsy, 188–196
    differential diagnosis of, 28, 189
Skew deviation, 184–187
Snellen eye chart, 1
Sphenoidal mucocele, optic neuritis vs, 38
Superior oblique palsy. See Fourth nerve palsy.
Sylvian aqueduct syndrome, 180
Sympathetic pupillary pathway, anatomy of, 32
Synkinetic facial movements, 257
Syphilis, optic nerve in, 118

Temporal arteritis. See Giant cell arteritis.
Temporal artery biopsy, in giant cell arteritis, 55
Temporal crescent, definition of, 9
Temporal lobe lesions
    homonymous hemianopia from, 23–24, 142–143
    localization of, 14
Tensilon test, 223–224

Third nerve palsy, 168–178
    aberrant regeneration with, 170–171, 174–175
    aneurysm causing, 172
    in cavernous sinus aneurysm, 176–177
    ischemic, 171, 173–174
    limited upgaze in, 158–159
    pupil sparing in, 171–172
Thyroid ophthalmopathy. See Graves' ophthalmopathy.
Tobacco-alcohol amblyopia, 92–94
Tolosa-Hunt syndrome, 218–220
Transient visual loss. See Amaurosis fugax.
Traumatic chiasmal syndrome, 100
Traumatic optic neuropathy, 98–101
Trochlear nerve palsy. See Fourth nerve palsy.

Uhthoff's phenomenon, 36
Upgaze, limited, 28, 153–162
    in blowout fracture, 160
    in cavernous sinus mass, 158–159
    in Graves' ophthalmopathy, 153–158
    in myasthenia gravis, 161
    in third nerve palsy, 158–159
Uveitis, dilated pupil due to, 243

Visual acuity
    definition, 1
    evaluation of, 1–2
Visual field
    Amsler grid, 9
    confrontation techniques, 9–11
    evaluation of, 8–14
    interpretation principles for, 13–14
    perimetry, 12–13
    tangent screen, 13
    terminology, 8–9
Visual field defect
    anatomic localization of, 13–14
    chiasmal lesion causing, 20–21
    in optic nerve disorders, 14–16
Visual function, evaluation of, 1–14

Walleyed bilateral internuclear ophthalmoplegia, 202–203